The Quick and Easy
Mediterranean Diet Cookbook

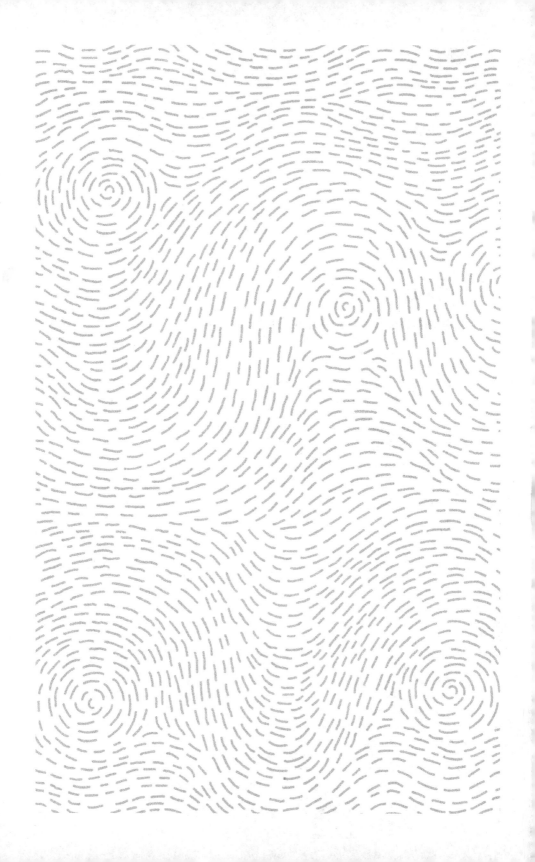

The Quick and Easy Mediterranean Diet Cookbook

76 MEDITERRANEAN DIET
RECIPES MADE IN MINUTES

ROCKRIDGE
PRESS

Contents

about the benefits of meal planning and doing some simple prep work before you begin cooking. In the remaining chapters, you will find more then seventy recipes that follow the principles of the diet.

The Mediterranean diet continues to grow in popularity, and after cooking from the flavorful and healthful recipes in these pages, you will understand why. With the help of this book, you will discover that the Mediterranean diet can be quick and easy!

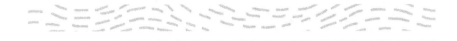

PART ONE

Getting Started

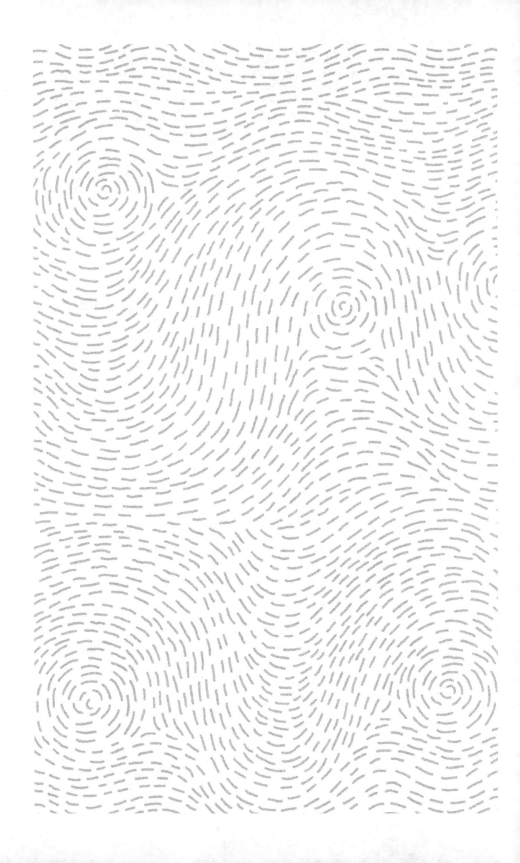

CHAPTER ONE

The Basics of the Mediterranean Diet

The Mediterranean diet is a lifestyle—including foods, activities, meals with friends and family, and wine in moderation with meals. It has been studied and noted by scores of leading scientists as one of the healthiest in the world. Just as important, the Mediterranean diet is full of wonderfully delicious, flavor-filled dishes and meals.

—Oldways Preservation Trust

WHAT IS THE MEDITERRANEAN DIET?

The goal of the Mediterranean diet is not weight loss, though you will probably shed some pounds. Instead, it is a lifestyle choice—a choice to engage in the healthful eating, portion control, and regular exercise that for centuries has been typical of the people living in the Mediterranean region. They consume whole grains that have been minimally processed, fresh fruits and vegetables, cheese and yogurt, seafood, and plenty of herbs and spices. Many dishes are cooked in or drizzled with olive oil.

- Saturated fats, such as butter
- Sugary sweets and candies

Now that you understand what the Mediterranean diet is and how it can benefit you, it's time to move on to more practical details. In the next chapter, you will learn some tips for saving your valuable time and money while following the Mediterranean diet.

CHAPTER TWO

How to Save Time and Money

Traditional Mediterranean meals feature foods grown all around the Mediterranean Sea and enjoyed along with lifestyle factors typical of this region. [These foods] are easily adaptable to today's kitchens and busy lives.

—Oldways Preservation Trust

For many people, following a diet can be an exasperating experience. Not only do you have to deal with food restrictions and reduced calorie counts, you may also find yourself eating the same things day after day. The Mediterranean diet eliminates those feelings of deprivation and dissatisfaction, and it ensures that you have plenty of meal options to choose from. One day you may be dining on a fresh cut of fish with tender vegetables, and the next day you may be digging into a bowl of hearty stew. The key to sticking to the Mediterranean diet is to choose foods you enjoy eating, and this book will help make that possible. In this chapter you will learn how planning ahead can help you save both time and money while following the Mediterranean diet.

PLANNING, SHOPPING, AND COOKING

When you are feeling good, it isn't hard to stick to your diet. If you are stressed about the time and money it takes to cook, however, you may feel less motivated. That is why it is so important to incorporate simple preparation tips and meal planning into the Mediterranean diet. Use the following steps to make the most of your time and money:

1. Go through the recipes in this book and pick out some that you'd like to try. When making your choices, consider which vegetables and seafood are in season in your region.
2. Make a list of recipes you want to prepare during the week. Try to include a variety of different dishes. If they have a few ingredients in common, you can save money and prep time.
3. Don't hesitate to clip coupons and search out sales! If you find yourself buying some things on a regular basis, check the weekly ads and buy extra when they're on sale.
4. Transfer your list of recipes to a weekly calendar, assigning one recipe to each meal for a week.
5. Create your shopping list by going through the ingredients lists in the recipes to determine what you need to buy.

According to a study conducted by the College of Human Ecology at Cornell University, sharing meals as a family can have a significant impact on the well-being of your children. The study revealed that regular family meals helped to reduce the likelihood that a child would engage in disordered eating by 35 percent, and the child was 12 percent less likely to become overweight. The benefits of sharing family dinners are undeniable, and engaging in simple meal-planning strategies can help to make it a reality for your family.

6. Do all of your shopping in one day, and store everything well so it will last until you need it.
7. Prepare some of the ingredients ahead of time, if possible. You can rinse and chop vegetables, trim cuts of meat, and remove shells from shrimp.
8. Follow the meal plan you created, preparing the meals you chose for each day of the week.
9. Make notes as you prepare each recipe, writing down tips you learned that will save you time when you make the same dish again.

By following these simple steps, you can save a great deal of time and money while following the Mediterranean diet. Having a weekly meal plan eliminates much of the stress of cooking, because you already know what you are going to make before you even get home. And you also already have the ingredients you need! Planning ahead also enables you to take advantage of seasonal produce at your local farmers' market. Before you know it, you will be planning your meals with ease, arranging them so the leftovers from one meal can be used as an ingredient in the next!

SIMPLE COOKING TIPS

Here are a few tips that should come in handy, whether you are an experienced cook or a complete novice:

- Don't feel like you need to purchase every kitchen appliance out there—often you can use a food processor instead of an immersion blender, or a blender instead of a food processor.
- Experiment with different herbs and spices. Mediterranean foods are never short on flavor, so don't be afraid to spice it up!
- Remember that although cooking with olive oil is healthier than using butter, olive oil is still high in calories. Use what you need, but don't overdo it!
- Greek yogurt makes a great substitute for heavy cream and sour cream in recipes—it gives your dish a smooth texture without all the added fat.
- Slow cooking is a great way to turn inexpensive, tougher cuts of meat into tender and flavorful dishes; the meat literally cooks in its own juices.
- Get fancy with the garnish! Topping even the simplest dish with a pinch of fresh herbs or a little grated lemon zest can add a new level of presentation.
- Don't be afraid to sip a glass of wine while cooking or enjoying your meal—you might even want to add a splash to your dish for flavor.

Now that you understand the basics and benefits of the Mediterranean diet, you are ready to try it for yourself! In the following pages you will find over seventy recipes, including breakfast items, soups and stews, salads, entrées, and even desserts.

You may turn your nose up at clipping coupons for fear that your favorite supermarket manager will think you've fallen on hard times. But this economical practice is more common than you might think. According to a survey conducted by Nielsen in 2009, nearly 20 percent of coupon users have an annual income of $100,000 or more. In fact, the top three income brackets in the survey showed the highest number of individuals who labeled themselves coupon "enthusiasts."

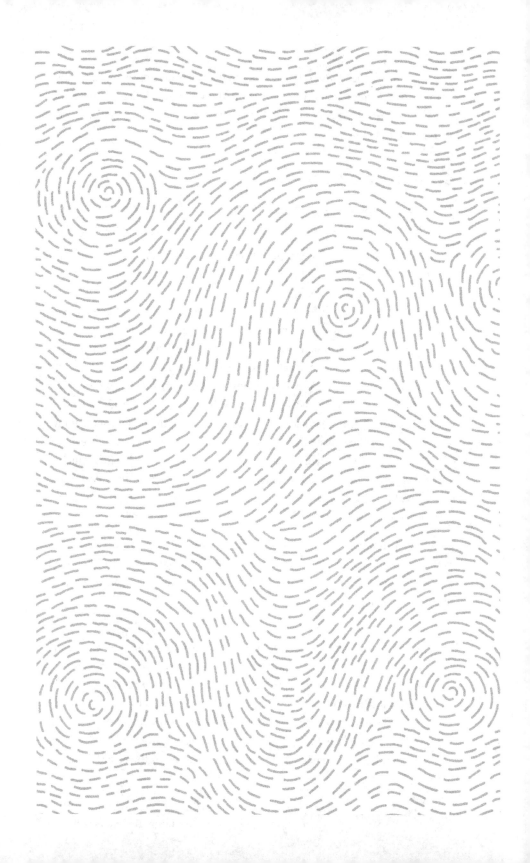

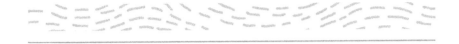

PART TWO

Quick and Easy Recipes

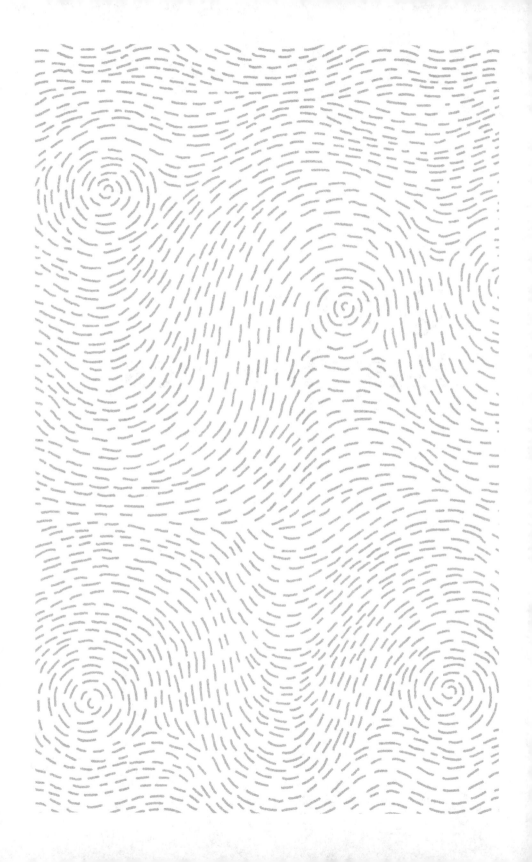

CHAPTER THREE

Breakfast

Spinach and Feta Omelet

SERVES 1

▶ PREP TIME: 5 MINUTES
▶ COOK TIME: 10 MINUTES

An omelet is a great way to start the day. It only takes a few minutes to prepare, but the fiber and protein will keep you feeling satisfied all morning long.

2 EGGS

1 TABLESPOON SKIM MILK

½ TEASPOON SALT

¼ TEASPOON BLACK PEPPER

2 TEASPOONS EXTRA-VIRGIN OLIVE OIL

1 CUP CHOPPED BABY SPINACH

2 TABLESPOONS CRUMBLED FETA CHEESE

2 TABLESPOONS SLICED GREEN ONION

1. Whisk the eggs, milk, salt, and pepper together in a small bowl and set aside.

2. Heat 1 teaspoon of the olive oil in a small nonstick skillet over medium heat. Add the spinach and stir to coat with oil. Cook for 1 to 2 minutes, until just wilted. Transfer the spinach to a small bowl and set aside.

3. Heat the remaining teaspoon of oil in the skillet. Pour in the egg mixture and cook for 1 minute without disturbing. Tilt the pan to spread out the uncooked egg and cook for 1 minute longer.

4. Use a spatula to scrape down the sides of the pan and cook until the eggs are almost set, about 1 minute more. Spoon the spinach over half the omelet and sprinkle with feta cheese.

5. Fold the empty half of the omelet over the filling to cover. Cook for 30 to 60 seconds, until the egg is set and the cheese is melted.

6. Slide the omelet onto a plate, garnish with green onion, and serve.

Tomato and Green Onion Omelet

SERVES 1

▶ PREP TIME: 5 MINUTES
▶ COOK TIME: 10 MINUTES

To get the most out of this tomato and green onion omelet, use fresh tomatoes from your own garden or from your local farmers' market.

2 EGGS
1 TABLESPOON SKIM MILK
½ TEASPOON SALT
¼ TEASPOON BLACK PEPPER
2 TEASPOONS EXTRA-VIRGIN OLIVE OIL
1 PLUM TOMATO, DICED
¼ CUP THINLY SLICED GREEN ONION

1. Whisk the eggs, milk, salt, and pepper together in a small bowl and set aside.

2. Heat 1 teaspoon of the olive oil in a small nonstick skillet over medium heat. Add the tomato and half the green onions and stir to coat with oil. Cook for 1 to 2 minutes, until just wilted.

3. Spoon the tomato and green onion mixture into a bowl, and heat the remaining teaspoon of oil in the skillet.

4. Pour in the egg mixture and cook, undisturbed, for 1 minute. Tilt the pan to spread out the uncooked egg and cook for 1 minute longer.

5. Use a spatula to scrape down the sides of the pan; then cook until the eggs are almost set, about 1 minute more. Spoon the tomato and green onion mixture over half the omelet.

6. Fold the empty half of the omelet over the filling. Cook for 30 to 60 seconds, until the egg is set.

7. Slide the omelet onto a plate, garnish with the remaining green onion, and serve.

Zucchini Onion Frittata

▶ PREP TIME: 10 MINUTES
▶ COOK TIME: 15 MINUTES

If you are cooking for your family or friends, or you simply want some leftovers for yourself, a big, hearty frittata is definitely the way to go. This savory version makes breakfast for a crowd.

2 TEASPOONS EXTRA-VIRGIN OLIVE OIL
1 GARLIC CLOVE, MINCED
2 CUPS SLICED ZUCCHINI
½ CUP CHOPPED ONION
½ TEASPOON SALT
¼ TEASPOON BLACK PEPPER
8 EGGS

1. Preheat the broiler to high.

2. Heat the olive oil in an ovenproof skillet with a lid over medium-high heat. Add the garlic and cook for 1 minute.

3. Stir in the zucchini and onion and season with salt and pepper. Cook for 4 to 5 minutes, stirring often, until the onions are translucent.

4. Beat the eggs in a bowl and pour into the skillet, stirring just until combined with the zucchini and onion. Cover, reduce the heat to low, and cook for 12 minutes, or until the egg are almost set.

5. Place the skillet under the broiler, uncovered, for 2 minutes, or until the eggs are lightly browned.

6. Let the frittata cool for 5 minutes, cut into portions, and serve.

Herbed Mushroom Frittata

SERVES 6

▶ PREP TIME: 10 MINUTES
▶ COOK TIME: 15 MINUTES

This frittata is a snap to throw together. In no time you have a hearty meal for the whole family.

2 TEASPOONS EXTRA-VIRGIN OLIVE OIL

1 GARLIC CLOVE, MINCED

2 CUPS DICED PORTOBELLO MUSHROOM

¼ CUP DICED RED ONION

½ TEASPOON SALT

¼ TEASPOON BLACK PEPPER

½ TEASPOON DRIED OREGANO

½ TEASPOON DRIED BASIL

8 EGGS

1. Preheat the broiler to high heat.

2. Heat the olive oil in an ovenproof skillet with a lid over medium-high heat. Add the garlic and cook for 1 minute.

3. Stir in the mushroom and onion, and season with the salt and pepper. Cook for 4 to 5 minutes, stirring often, until the onions are translucent. Stir in the oregano and basil.

4. Beat the eggs in a bowl and pour into the skillet, stirring just until combined with the mushroom and onions. Cover, reduce the heat to low, and cook for 12 minutes, or until the egg is almost set.

5. Place the skillet under the broiler, uncovered, for 2 minutes, or until the eggs are lightly browned.

6. Let the frittata cool for 5 minutes, cut into portions, and serve.

Cherry and Almond Oatmeal

SERVES 4

▶ PREP TIME: 5 MINUTES
▶ COOK TIME: 10 MINUTES

Instant oatmeal packets have nothing on this recipe. There is just something about the combination of freshly cooked oats, tart cherries, and almonds that pleases the palate. Here, they come together in a snap. For this recipe and the one that follows, make sure you use quick-cooking steel-cut oats. Instant oats have a bland flavor and little nutritional value, and regular steel-cut oats take four times as long to cook!

3 CUPS WATER
1 CUP QUICK-COOKING STEEL-CUT OATS
⅓ CUP DRIED TART CHERRIES
1 TABLESPOON HONEY
¼ TEASPOON GROUND CINNAMON
PINCH OF SALT
¼ CUP THINLY SLICED ALMONDS

1. Bring the water to a boil in a medium saucepan over medium-high heat.

2. Whisk in the oats, cherries, honey, cinnamon, and salt.

3. Reduce the heat to low and simmer the mixture, uncovered, for about 5 minutes, or until the oats are tender. For a creamier texture, stir oatmeal constantly during cooking.

4. Spoon the oatmeal into bowls and sprinkle with sliced almonds to serve.

Cinnamon Pumpkin Oatmeal

SERVES 4

▶ PREP TIME: 5 MINUTES
▶ COOK TIME: 15 MINUTES

Pumpkin and cinnamon are simply meant to be together. Here, they join oatmeal for a homey, satisfying breakfast.

3 CUPS WATER

1 CUP QUICK-COOKING STEEL-CUT OATS

2 TABLESPOONS PUMPKIN PURÉE

1 TABLESPOON HONEY

¼ TEASPOON PUMPKIN PIE SPICE

PINCH OF SALT

1. Bring the water to a boil in a medium saucepan over medium-high heat.

2. Whisk in the oats, pumpkin purée, honey, pumpkin pie spice, and salt.

3. Reduce the heat to low and simmer the mixture, uncovered, for about 5 minutes, or until the oats are tender. For a creamier texture, stir oatmeal constantly during cooking.

4. Spoon the oatmeal into bowls and serve.

Maple Cinnamon Couscous

SERVES 4

▶ PREP TIME: 5 MINUTES
▶ COOK TIME: 15 MINUTES

Couscous is more than just a side dish. This recipe proves that, with the right seasoning, it can become a tasty breakfast treat! Feel free to substitute water, soy milk, or almond milk for part or all of the milk.

2½ CUPS SKIM MILK
2 TEASPOONS GROUND CINNAMON
1 CUP WHOLE-WHEAT COUSCOUS, UNCOOKED
2 TABLESPOONS PURE MAPLE SYRUP
¼ TEASPOON VANILLA EXTRACT
PINCH OF SALT

1. Heat the milk and cinnamon in a medium saucepan over medium-high heat until bubbles begin to form around the edges of the milk.

2. Remove from heat and stir in the couscous, maple syrup, vanilla, and salt.

3. Cover and let stand for 5 to 10 minutes, until the couscous absorbs the milk.

4. Fluff the couscous with a fork, spoon into bowls, and serve.

Honey Walnut Couscous

SERVES 4

▶ PREP TIME: 5 MINUTES
▶ COOK TIME: 15 MINUTES

This couscous is hot and hearty—just what you need for a satisfying breakfast. The walnuts lend a little crunch. Substitute water, soy milk, or almond milk for part or all of the milk if you prefer.

2½ CUPS SKIM MILK
½ TEASPOON GROUND CINNAMON
¼ TEASPOON GROUND NUTMEG
1 CUP WHOLE-WHEAT COUSCOUS, UNCOOKED
2 TABLESPOONS HONEY
¼ TEASPOON VANILLA EXTRACT
PINCH OF SALT
¼ CUP CHOPPED WALNUTS

1. Heat the milk, cinnamon, and nutmeg in a medium saucepan over medium-high heat until bubbles begin to form around the edges.

2. Remove from the heat and stir in the couscous, honey, vanilla extract, and salt.

3. Cover and let stand for 5 to 10 minutes, until the couscous absorbs the milk.

4. Fluff the couscous with a fork and spoon into bowls to serve. Garnish with chopped walnuts.

Sweet Banana Pancakes

SERVES 2

▶ PREP TIME: 5 MINUTES

▶ COOK TIME: 10 MINUTES

These banana pancakes are so simple to prepare and only require three ingredients. They're also wheat-free, suitable for those who need to avoid gluten.

4 EGGS

3 RIPE BANANAS

¼ TEASPOON BAKING POWDER

1. Crack the eggs into a medium mixing bowl and beat well. In another medium bowl, mash the bananas with a potato masher. Add the eggs and baking powder to the bananas and stir until blended well.

2. Heat a large nonstick skillet over medium-low heat. Spoon the batter onto the skillet, using 1 to 2 tablespoons per pancake.

3. Cook the pancakes for 1 to 2 minutes on the first side, until bubbles begin to form on the surface. Carefully flip the pancakes and cook for 1 minute more, until lightly browned on the underside.

4. Transfer the pancakes to a serving plate and tent with foil to keep warm. Repeat with the remaining batter.

Easy Blueberry Pancakes

SERVES 3

▶ PREP TIME: 5 MINUTES

▶ COOK TIME: 15 MINUTES

These blueberry pancakes are light and fluffy, and they are made without oil or sugar. The secret? Greek yogurt!

1½ CUPS PLAIN GREEK YOGURT

2 EGGS

2 TABLESPOONS AGAVE NECTAR

1 CUP ALL-PURPOSE FLOUR

2 TEASPOONS BAKING SODA

PINCH OF SALT

COOKING SPRAY (OPTIONAL)

1 CUP FRESH BLUEBERRIES

1. Beat together the yogurt, eggs, and agave nectar in a medium mixing bowl.

2. In a small bowl, whisk together the flour, baking soda, and salt. Add this mixture to the wet ingredients and whisk until just combined and free of lumps.

3. Heat a large nonstick skillet over medium heat. Coat it with cooking spray, if needed.

4. For each pancake, spoon about ¼ cup of batter into the skillet and drop a few blueberries into the wet batter. Cook the pancakes for about 2 minutes on the first side, or until browned. Carefully flip the pancakes and cook for another 2 minutes or until lightly browned underneath.

5. Transfer the cooked pancakes to a serving plate and tent with foil to keep warm. Repeat with the remaining batter.

Whole-Wheat Muffins

MAKES 24 MINI MUFFINS

▶ PREP TIME: 10 MINUTES
▶ COOK TIME: 15 MINUTES

Made with whole-wheat flour and rolled oats, these muffins are much healthier than anything that comes from a box.

1 CUP WHOLE-WHEAT FLOUR
1 CUP ROLLED (OLD-FASHIONED) OATS
1 TEASPOON BAKING SODA
½ TEASPOON GROUND NUTMEG
¼ TEASPOON SALT
1 CUP UNSWEETENED APPLESAUCE
½ CUP PURE MAPLE SYRUP
2 EGGS
1 TEASPOON VANILLA EXTRACT

1. Preheat the oven to 325°F and line a 24-cup mini muffin pan with paper liners.

2. Combine the flour, oats, baking soda, nutmeg, and salt in a medium bowl.

3. Whisk together the applesauce, maple syrup, eggs, and vanilla in a large mixing bowl until well combined. Add the flour mixture in small batches and beat until just combined.

4. Spoon the batter into the muffin cups, filling each one almost to the top. Bake for 15 minutes, or so until the tip of a knife inserted in the center comes out clean.

5. Cool the muffins in the pan for 5 minutes; then turn them out onto wire racks to cool completely.

Cinnamon Raisin Muffins

MAKES 24 MINI MUFFINS

- ▶ PREP TIME: 10 MINUTES
- ▶ COOK TIME: 15 MINUTES

The smell of these cinnamon raisin muffins is sure to get even the deepest sleepers out of bed for breakfast in the morning.

1 CUP WHOLE-WHEAT FLOUR

1 CUP ROLLED (OLD-FASHIONED) OATS

1 TEASPOON BAKING SODA

1½ TEASPOONS GROUND CINNAMON

¼ TEASPOON SALT

1 CUP UNSWEETENED APPLESAUCE

½ CUP RAW HONEY

2 EGGS

1 TEASPOON VANILLA EXTRACT

¾ CUP RAISINS

1. Preheat oven to 325°F and line a 24-cup mini muffin pan with paper liners.

2. Combine the flour, oats, baking soda, cinnamon, and salt in a medium bowl.

3. Whisk together the applesauce, honey, eggs, and vanilla in a large mixing bowl until well combined. Add the flour mixture in small batches and beat until just combined. Fold in the raisins.

4. Spoon the batter into the muffin cups, filling them almost to the top. Bake for 15 minutes or until the point of a knife inserted in the center comes out clean.

5. Cool the muffins in the pan for 5 minutes, and then turn them out onto wire racks to cool completely.

Almond and Banana Smoothie

SERVES 2

▶ PREP TIME: 5 MINUTES

Almonds are a great source of protein and heart-healthy fats. In this recipe, their flavor blends well with the slight sweetness of banana.

2 BANANAS, FROZEN AND SLICED

1 CUP COLD UNSWEETENED ALMOND MILK

½ CUP PLAIN GREEK YOGURT

3 TABLESPOONS RAW ALMONDS

1 TEASPOON HONEY

1. Combine all of the ingredients in a blender.

2. Blend on high speed for 30 to 60 seconds, until smooth and well combined.

3. Pour into two glasses and serve immediately.

Strawberry and Hemp Smoothie

▶ PREP TIME: 5 MINUTES

Hemp seed is a good source of both vegetarian protein and fiber. When combined with frozen strawberries, which are rich in potassium, the result is a smoothie with a powerful nutritional punch.

2 CUPS FROZEN SLICED STRAWBERRIES
1 CUP COLD UNSWEETENED ALMOND MILK
½ CUP PLAIN GREEK YOGURT
2 TABLESPOONS GROUND HEMP SEED
1 TEASPOON HONEY

1. Combine all of the ingredients in a blender.

2. Blend on high speed for 30 to 60 seconds, until smooth and well combined.

3. Pour into two glasses and serve immediately.

Blueberry Yogurt Smoothie

SERVES 2

▶ PREP TIME: 5 MINUTES

The blueberries in this smoothie are loaded with antioxidants, while the Greek yogurt gives you a morning protein boost.

2 CUPS FROZEN BLUEBERRIES
1 CUP COLD UNSWEETENED ALMOND MILK
1 CUP PLAIN GREEK YOGURT
1 TEASPOON HONEY

1. Combine all of the ingredients in a blender.

2. Blend on high speed for 30 to 60 seconds, until smooth and well combined.

3. Pour into two glasses and serve immediately.

Cranberry and Banana Smoothie

SERVES 2

▶ PREP TIME: 5 MINUTES

This smoothie is nice and light. The cranberries balance the banana nicely, and together they'll brighten your morning.

2 BANANAS, FROZEN AND SLICED

1 CUP FROZEN CRANBERRIES

1 CUP COLD VANILLA ALMOND MILK

¼ CUP UNSWEETENED CRANBERRY JUICE

¼ CUP PLAIN GREEK YOGURT

2 TABLESPOONS HONEY

1. Combine all of the ingredients in a blender.

2. Blend on high speed for 30 to 60 seconds, until smooth and well combined.

3. Pour into two glasses and serve immediately.

Apricot Blueberry Smoothie

▶ PREP TIME: 5 MINUTES

This creamy and refreshing smoothie blends the tartness of apricot juice with the sweetness of blueberries. Together they'll bring a zippy start to your day.

2 CUPS FROZEN BLUEBERRIES

½ CUP COLD APRICOT JUICE

½ CUP COLD VANILLA ALMOND MILK

¼ CUP PLAIN GREEK YOGURT

1 TABLESPOON HONEY

1. Combine all of the ingredients in a blender.

2. Blend on high speed for 30 to 60 seconds, until smooth and well combined.

3. Pour into two glasses and serve immediately.

Orange and Pomegranate Smoothie

SERVES 2

▶ PREP TIME: 5 MINUTES

Pomegranates are filled with antioxidants, which stop the cellular damage caused by free radicals. (Free radicals are themselves damaged, and dangerous, molecules.) Antioxidants can also help prevent cancer and other chronic diseases.

1 CUP COLD UNSWEETENED POMEGRANATE JUICE
1 CUP COLD VANILLA ALMOND MILK
1 CUP FROZEN SLICED PEACHES
1 NAVEL ORANGE, PEELED AND SECTIONED
2 TABLESPOONS HONEY

1. Combine all of the ingredients in a blender.

2. Blend on high speed for 30 to 60 seconds, until smooth and well combined.

3. Pour into two glasses and serve immediately.

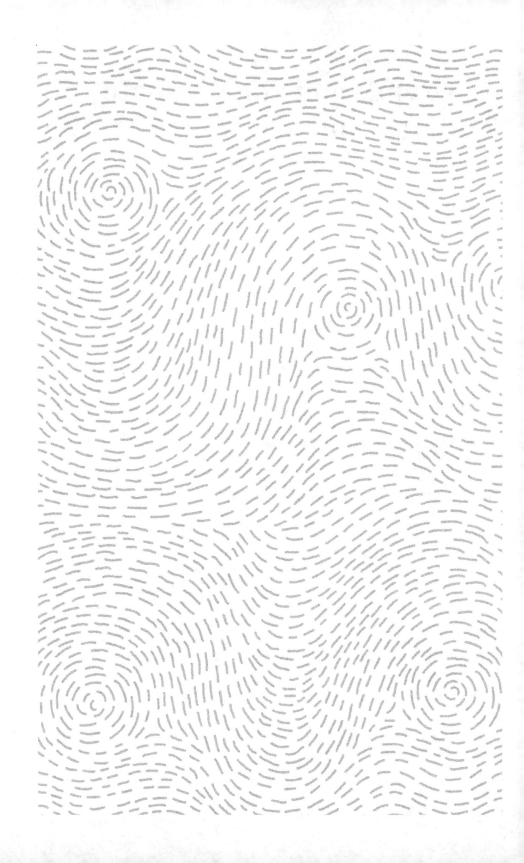

CHAPTER FOUR

Appetizers and Snacks

Tomato and Almond Pesto

MAKES ABOUT 4 CUPS

▶ PREP TIME: 15 MINUTES

This tomato and almond pesto is a unique twist on traditional basil pesto. Made with a mix of fire-roasted and plain tomatoes and toasted almonds instead of pine nuts, it retains a distinctly Mediterranean flavor. Serve it with toasted pita bread.

¾ CUP SLIVERED ALMONDS
ONE 28-OUNCE CAN DICED TOMATOES, DRAINED
ONE 14-OUNCE CAN FIRE-ROASTED TOMATOES, DRAINED
1 CUP FRESH BASIL LEAVES
1 TABLESPOON RED WINE VINEGAR
¾ CUP EXTRA-VIRGIN OLIVE OIL
½ CUP GRATED PARMESAN CHEESE
SALT AND PEPPER TO TASTE

1. Heat a large skillet over medium-high heat and add the almonds. Toast the almonds for 3 to 5 minutes in the dry pan, stirring often, until golden.

2. Transfer the almonds to a food processor and process until ground into a fine powder.

3. Add all the tomatoes, the basil, and red wine vinegar. Blend until smooth. With the food processor running, pour in the olive oil slowly. Blend for 30 seconds. Add the Parmesan cheese, salt, and pepper, and pulse several times to combine.

4. Serve at room temperature or chill until ready to serve.

Roasted Eggplant Feta Dip

SERVES 10 TO 12

▶ PREP TIME: 10 MINUTES
▶ COOK TIME: 15 MINUTES

This hearty dip goes perfectly with slices of warm pita bread. Herb-Tossed Olives (page 43) would make a nice companion dish.

1 EGGPLANT
2 TABLESPOONS LEMON JUICE
¼ CUP EXTRA-VIRGIN OLIVE OIL
¼ CUP DICED RED ONION
½ CUP DICED RED BELL PEPPER
1 JALAPEÑO PEPPER, SEEDED AND MINCED
2 TABLESPOONS CHOPPED FRESH BASIL
1 TABLESPOON CHOPPED FRESH CHIVES
½ CUP CRUMBLED FETA CHEESE
SALT AND PEPPER TO TASTE

1. Preheat the broiler and line a baking sheet with foil.

2. Using a sharp knife, make small slits in the flesh of the eggplant to vent steam while it roasts. Place the eggplant on the baking sheet.

3. Roast the eggplant, turning it every 5 minutes, until the flesh pierces easily with a knife, about 15 minutes. Transfer to a cutting board and let sit until cool enough to handle.

4. Cut the eggplant in half and spoon the tender flesh into a medium bowl. Add the lemon juice and then the remaining ingredients, and stir until well combined. Serve warm.

Herbed Olive Oil Bread Dip

SERVES 4

▶ PREP TIME: 5 MINUTES

This herbed dipping oil is the perfect complement to a crusty loaf of whole-grain bread, which is a staple of the Mediterranean diet.

¼ CUP EXTRA-VIRGIN OLIVE OIL

1 TABLESPOON CHOPPED FRESH THYME

1 TABLESPOON CHOPPED FRESH CHIVES

1 TABLESPOON CHOPPED FRESH ROSEMARY

½ TEASPOON SEA SALT

FRESH BREAD, FOR SERVING

1. Combine the oil, herbs, and salt in a small bowl and stir together well.

2. Serve the oil at room temperature with slices of fresh bread for dipping.

Watermelon Gazpacho

SERVES 6

▶ PREP TIME: 10 MINUTES

Gazpacho is traditionally made with tomatoes, but here it is made with watermelon, flavored with a hint of lime. It's the perfect appetizer on a hot day.

8 CUPS CHOPPED SEEDLESS WATERMELON
1 SEEDLESS CUCUMBER, CHOPPED
2 CELERY STALKS, CHOPPED
2 RIPE TOMATOES, CHOPPED
1 TEASPOON MINCED GARLIC
3 TABLESPOONS FRESH LIME JUICE
2 TABLESPOONS RICE VINEGAR
2 TABLESPOONS CHOPPED FRESH CILANTRO
1 TABLESPOON CHOPPED FRESH BASIL
SALT

1. Set aside 1 cup of chopped watermelon and place the rest in a food processor.

2. Add the cucumber, celery, tomatoes, and garlic. Pulse several times until finely chopped but not quite puréed.

3. Transfer to a large bowl and whisk in the lime juice, vinegar, herbs, and salt.

4. Pour the soup into a storage container and stir in the reserved watermelon.

5. Cover and refrigerate for at least 2 hours. Serve chilled.

Easy Antipasto Salad

SERVES 8

▶ PREP TIME: 15 MINUTES

Antipasto salad is an iconic Mediterranean recipe that can be enjoyed as an appetizer, first course, or entrée.

2 HEARTS OF ROMAINE LETTUCE, CHOPPED

1 CUP PACKED PARSLEY LEAVES, CHOPPED

ONE 8-OUNCE JAR ROASTED RED PEPPERS, DRAINED AND CHOPPED

TWO 6-OUNCE JARS ARTICHOKE HEARTS, DRAINED AND CHOPPED

1 CUP ASSORTED PITTED OLIVES, DRAINED

1 CUP PEPPERONCINI, DRAINED

4 CUPS CHERRY TOMATOES, HALVED

1 RED ONION, HALVED AND THINLY SLICED

VINAIGRETTE

⅓ CUP EXTRA-VIRGIN OLIVE OIL

3 TABLESPOONS RED WINE VINEGAR

1 GARLIC CLOVE, MINCED

½ TEASPOON SUGAR

PINCH OF SALT AND PEPPER

1. Spread out the romaine in a layer on a large platter and top with parsley, roasted red peppers, artichokes, olives, pepperoncini, tomatoes, and onion.

2. To make the vinaigrette, whisk together the olive oil, vinegar, garlic, sugar, salt, and pepper.

3. Drizzle the vinaigrette over the salad and serve immediately.

Cool Cucumber Salad

SERVES 6

▶ PREP TIME: 15 MINUTES

This cool cucumber salad is light and refreshing. It makes a quick and easy first course or snack—just what you need on a hot day!

1 LARGE SEEDLESS CUCUMBER, PEELED AND CHOPPED

2 SMALL PICKLING CUCUMBERS, THINLY SLICED

½ RED ONION, DICED

1 HEIRLOOM TOMATO, SEEDED AND DICED

DRESSING

¼ CUP WHITE WINE VINEGAR

1 TABLESPOON BALSAMIC VINEGAR

1 TABLESPOON EXTRA-VIRGIN OLIVE OIL

2 TEASPOONS HONEY

SALT AND PEPPER TO TASTE

1. Combine the chopped and sliced cucumbers, onion, and tomato in a large bowl. Toss well.

2. To make the dressing, whisk together the vinegars, olive oil, honey, salt, and pepper in a small bowl.

3. Pour dressing over the salad, toss to coat, and refrigerate until ready to serve.

Caprese Salad

SERVES 4

▶ PREP TIME: 10 MINUTES

A caprese salad is a refreshing combination of ripe tomatoes, fresh mozzarella, and basil leaves, attractively arranged on a plate.

3 RIPE HEIRLOOM TOMATOES, THINLY SLICED
ONE 8-OUNCE BALL FRESH MOZZARELLA, SLICED THIN
1 BUNCH FRESH BASIL
SALT AND PEPPER TO TASTE
2 TABLESPOONS EXTRA-VIRGIN OLIVE OIL
1 TABLESPOON BALSAMIC VINEGAR

1. Arrange the tomato and mozzarella slices on a platter, alternating between the two and overlapping them slightly.

2. Tuck the fresh basil leaves between the mozzarella and tomato slices, and season with salt and pepper.

3. Whisk together the olive oil and balsamic vinegar, drizzle over the salad, and serve.

Herb-Tossed Olives

SERVES 4

▶ PREP TIME: 10 MINUTES

Serve these savory olives in small bowls at your next dinner party. People love snacking on this quintessentially Mediterranean food.

3 CUPS ASSORTED PITTED OLIVES
2 TEASPOONS EXTRA-VIRGIN OLIVE OIL
⅛ TEASPOON DRIED OREGANO
⅛ TEASPOON DRIED THYME
⅛ TEASPOON DRIED BASIL
1 GARLIC CLOVE, CRUSHED
BLACK PEPPER TO TASTE

1. Place the olives in a medium bowl and drizzle with the olive oil.

2. Add the herbs and garlic and season with pepper.

3. Toss the mixture to combine and chill until ready to serve.

Marinated Olives with Feta

▶ PREP TIME: 10 MINUTES

Rich in flavor, these olives are incredibly easy to put together. You may want to keep a bowl in the refrigerator at all times for snacking!

2 CUPS PITTED KALAMATA OLIVES, DRAINED AND SLICED
½ CUP CRUMBLED FETA CHEESE
2 TABLESPOONS EXTRA-VIRGIN OLIVE OIL
2 TABLESPOONS LEMON JUICE
2 GARLIC CLOVES, MINCED
1 TEASPOON GRATED LEMON ZEST
BLACK PEPPER TO TASTE

1. Place the olives in a medium bowl and toss with the feta cheese and olive oil.

2. Add the lemon juice, garlic, and lemon zest and mix well.

3. Season with pepper, and refrigerate until ready to serve.

Heirloom Tomato Basil Skewers

SERVES 4

▶ PREP TIME: 10 MINUTES

If you are looking for a quick and flavorful appetizer or snack, these festive tomato and basil skewers are just the thing.

2 CUPS HEIRLOOM CHERRY TOMATOES, HALVED

2 CUPS SMALL FRESH MOZZARELLA BALLS (*CILIEGINE*)

1 BUNCH FRESH BASIL

2 TABLESPOONS EXTRA-VIRGIN OLIVE OIL

SALT AND PEPPER TO TASTE

1. Thread 1 tomato half, 1 mozzarella ball, 1 basil leaf, and another tomato half on a wooden skewer or toothpick. Repeat with the remaining tomatoes, mozzarella, and basil.

2. Arrange the skewers on a tray. Drizzle with olive oil, season with salt and pepper, and serve.

Cucumber Mozzarella Skewers

▶ PREP TIME: 10 MINUTES

This recipe is a tasty twist on a traditional caprese salad, made with cucumbers instead of tomatoes. For the best flavor, take advantage of your local farmers' market and buy fresh cucumbers in season.

2 SEEDLESS CUCUMBERS, SLICED ¼ INCH THICK
ONE 8-OUNCE BALL FRESH MOZZARELLA, THINLY SLICED
1 BUNCH FRESH BASIL
2 TABLESPOONS EXTRA-VIRGIN OLIVE OIL
1 TABLESPOON BALSAMIC VINEGAR
SALT AND PEPPER TO TASTE

1. Arrange half the cucumber slices on a platter, and top each one with a slice of mozzarella and a basil leaf.

2. Top the mozzarella and basil with another slice of cucumber, and skewer with a toothpick.

3. Whisk together the olive oil and balsamic vinegar, and season with salt and pepper to taste. Drizzle over the cucumber skewers and serve.

CHAPTER FIVE

Soups and Salads

Creamy Celery Soup

SERVES 4

▶ PREP TIME: 10 MINUTES
▶ COOK TIME: 15 MINUTES

Celery is known for its anti-inflammatory benefits, and it has also been shown to support digestive and cardiovascular health. Though coconut milk is not a traditionally Mediterranean ingredient, its light creamy flavor and healthy nutritional profile make it an excellent fit. Unsweetened soy milk, almond milk, or skim milk would also work in this recipe.

1 TABLESPOON EXTRA-VIRGIN OLIVE OIL
1 TEASPOON MINCED GARLIC
½ CUP DICED ONION
6 CELERY STALKS, DICED
1 YUKON GOLD POTATO, PEELED AND DICED
4 CUPS VEGETABLE BROTH
1 CUP UNSWEETENED COCONUT MILK
SALT AND PEPPER TO TASTE

1. Heat the olive oil in a large soup pot over medium-high heat. Add the garlic, onion, and celery and cook for 3 minutes, stirring.

2. Stir in the potato and vegetable broth and bring to a simmer. Lower the heat and simmer, covered, for 15 minutes, or until the celery and potato are very tender.

3. Remove from the heat and purée the soup with an immersion blender, or in batches in a traditional blender.

4. Whisk in the coconut milk, season with salt and pepper, and warm until the soup is hot.

Curried Carrot and Sweet Potato Soup

SERVES 4

▶ PREP TIME: 15 MINUTES
▶ COOK TIME: 15 MINUTES

This creamy soup has just a hint of curry to complement the cooked carrots and sweet potato. Carrots are a great source of vitamin A.

1 TABLESPOON EXTRA-VIRGIN OLIVE OIL
1 TEASPOON MINCED GARLIC
1 ONION, CHOPPED
2 CUPS GRATED CARROT
1 SWEET POTATO, PEELED AND GRATED
4 CUPS VEGETABLE BROTH
1 TEASPOON CURRY POWDER
SALT AND PEPPER TO TASTE

1. Heat the olive oil in a large soup pot over medium-high heat. Add the garlic and onion and cook for 3 minutes, stirring.

2. Stir in the carrot, sweet potato, vegetable broth, and curry powder, and season with salt and pepper.

3. Bring to a simmer, lower the heat, and cook, covered, for 15 minutes, or until the carrot and sweet potato are very tender.

4. Remove from the heat and purée the soup with an immersion blender, or in batches in a traditional blender. Adjust seasonings, if needed, and serve hot.

Butternut Squash Soup

SERVES 4

▶ PREP TIME: 10 MINUTES
▶ COOK TIME: 15 MINUTES

Butternut squash soup is a fall favorite, but you can make it all year round. Try this recipe and see how simple it is to make!

1 TABLESPOON EXTRA-VIRGIN OLIVE OIL
1 TEASPOON MINCED GARLIC
1 ONION, DICED
2 CELERY STALKS, DICED
2 TEASPOONS CURRY POWDER
4 CUPS DICED BUTTERNUT SQUASH
5 CUPS VEGETABLE BROTH
1 CUP UNSWEETENED COCONUT, SOY, ALMOND, OR SKIM MILK
SALT AND PEPPER TO TASTE

1. Heat the olive oil in a large soup pot over medium heat. Add the garlic and cook for 1 minute. Stir in the onion, celery, and curry powder and cook for 3 minutes, stirring.

2. Add the squash and broth and bring to a simmer. Lower the heat and cook, covered, for 15 minutes or until the squash is tender.

3. Remove from the heat and purée the soup with an immersion blender until smooth.

4. Whisk in the coconut milk and reheat the soup. Season with salt and pepper and serve.

Spiced Sweet Potato Soup

SERVES 6

▶ PREP TIME: 10 MINUTES
▶ COOK TIME: 15 MINUTES

This soup has a secret ingredient, puréed pumpkin, which adds to the creamy texture and slightly sweet flavor of the dish.

2 TABLESPOONS EXTRA-VIRGIN OLIVE OIL
1 TEASPOON MINCED GARLIC
1 ONION, DICED
4 CARROTS, PEELED AND CHOPPED
2 CELERY STALKS, CHOPPED
½ TEASPOON CURRY POWDER
¼ TEASPOON GROUND GINGER
SALT AND PEPPER TO TASTE
ONE 15-OUNCE CAN PUMPKIN PURÉE
1 SWEET POTATO, PEELED AND CUBED
6 CUPS VEGETABLE BROTH
2 TABLESPOONS DRY SHERRY

1. Heat the oil in a large soup pot over medium heat. Add the garlic and onion and cook for 3 minutes, stirring.

2. Add the carrots, celery, curry powder, ginger, salt and pepper, pumpkin purée, sweet potato, vegetable broth, and sherry. Stir well and bring to a simmer.

3. Lower the heat and simmer, covered, for 15 minutes or until the vegetables are tender.

4. Remove from heat and purée the soup with an immersion blender, or in batches in a traditional blender. Adjust the seasonings, if needed, and serve hot.

Roasted Vegetable Chowder

SERVES 6 TO 8

▶ PREP TIME: 15 MINUTES
▶ COOK TIME: 25 MINUTES

This blend of corn, tomatoes, sweet potato, and cauliflower is packed with nutrients as well as flavor.

1 ONION, CHOPPED

2 TABLESPOONS MINCED GARLIC

1 SWEET POTATO, PEELED AND CHOPPED

2 CARROTS, PEELED AND CHOPPED

2 CUPS CAULIFLOWER FLORETS

5 PLUM TOMATOES, CHOPPED

2 CUPS CORN KERNELS, FRESH OR FROZEN

2 TABLESPOONS EXTRA-VIRGIN OLIVE OIL

2 TEASPOONS DRIED THYME

SALT AND PEPPER TO TASTE

4 CUPS VEGETABLE BROTH

1 CUP UNSWEETENED COCONUT, SOY, ALMOND, OR SKIM MILK

1. Preheat the oven to 400°F.

2. To roast the vegetables, spread out the onion, garlic, sweet potato, carrots, cauliflower, tomatoes, and corn in a large baking pan. Toss together with the olive oil and dried thyme. Season with salt and pepper. Stir in about 1 cup of the vegetable broth and roast for 15 minutes or until tender, stirring once halfway through the roasting time.

3. Transfer the roasted veggies to a large soup pot, add the remaining 3 cups of broth, and bring to a simmer. Lower the heat and simmer, covered, for 10 minutes.

4. Remove from the heat and purée the soup with an immersion blender, or in batches in a traditional blender. Whisk in the coconut milk and adjust seasoning if necessary. Rewarm the soup and serve.

Spicy Chicken Chili

SERVES 6

▶ PREP TIME: 10 MINUTES
▶ COOK TIME: 15 MINUTES

This chili is easy to throw together, and it packs quite a punch! Serve it with pita chips.

1 TABLESPOON EXTRA-VIRGIN OLIVE OIL
1 TEASPOON MINCED GARLIC
2 CUPS CHOPPED BONELESS CHICKEN BREAST
1 CUP DICED ONION
2 JALAPEÑO PEPPERS, SEEDED AND MINCED
TWO 15-OUNCE CANS PINTO BEANS, RINSED AND DRAINED
ONE 28-OUNCE CAN FIRE-ROASTED TOMATOES, WITH THEIR JUICE
1 CUP DICED GREEN BELL PEPPER
2 CUPS CHICKEN BROTH
½ TEASPOON CAYENNE PEPPER
SALT AND PEPPER TO TASTE

1. Heat the olive oil in a Dutch oven over medium-high heat. Add the garlic and cook for 1 minute. Add the chicken and onion and cook, stirring, until the chicken is lightly browned, about 3 minutes.

2. Stir in the jalapeño peppers, beans, tomatoes, green pepper, and chicken broth and bring to a simmer.

3. Reduce the heat and simmer, covered, for 15 minutes or until the chicken is cooked through and the peppers are tender. Add cayenne pepper, season with salt and pepper, and serve.

Red Bean Sausage Stew

▶ PREP TIME: 10 MINUTES
▶ COOK TIME: 15 MINUTES

When you are looking for a spicy and hearty dish, keep this stew in mind. Serve it with rice. When combined with the beans, this will give you a complete protein.

2 TABLESPOONS CANOLA OIL

2 ANDOUILLE CHICKEN SAUSAGES, SLICED

1 RED ONION, DICED

1 TABLESPOON MINCED GARLIC

TWO 14-OUNCE CANS FIRE-ROASTED TOMATOES

THREE 15-OUNCE CANS RED KIDNEY BEANS, RINSED AND DRAINED

2½ CUPS CHICKEN BROTH

1 TABLESPOON APPLE CIDER VINEGAR

1 TEASPOON GROUND CUMIN

SALT AND PEPPER TO TASTE

1. Heat the oil in a Dutch oven over medium-high heat. Add the sausage, onion, and garlic and cook, stirring, until the onion is tender and the sausage is lightly browned, about 5 minutes.

2. Stir in the tomatoes, beans, broth, vinegar, cumin, salt, and pepper, and bring to a simmer. Reduce the heat and simmer, uncovered, for 15 minutes or until the flavors are well blended.

3. Ladle into bowls and serve.

Roasted Pepper Pasta Salad

SERVES 4

▶ PREP TIME: 15 MINUTES

This hearty whole-wheat pasta salad is tossed in a tangy dressing made with Greek yogurt and lemon juice.

6 OUNCES WHOLE-WHEAT PENNE

2 TABLESPOONS PLAIN GREEK YOGURT

⅔ CUP ROASTED RED PEPPERS

2 TABLESPOONS CHOPPED FRESH BASIL

1 TABLESPOON EXTRA-VIRGIN OLIVE OIL

1½ TEASPOONS FRESH LEMON JUICE

1 GARLIC CLOVE, MINCED

SALT AND PEPPER TO TASTE

½ CUP CHOPPED RED ONION

2 TABLESPOONS CAPERS, RINSED WELL

1. Bring a pot of salted water to boil. Cook the pasta according to the package directions until al dente. Drain, rinse in cool water, and drain again. Transfer to a large bowl.

2. Combine the yogurt, half the roasted red peppers, basil, olive oil, lemon juice, garlic, and salt and pepper in a food processor and process until smooth. Add to the pasta and toss.

3. Add the remaining red peppers, the onion, and capers and toss again.

4. Cover and chill until ready to serve.

Tomato Couscous Salad

▶ PREP TIME: 10 MINUTES

Couscous are grains of durum wheat, which are traditionally cooked with steam. In this recipe, cooked couscous is tossed with tomatoes and a vinaigrette dressing.

2 CUPS CHICKEN STOCK

ONE 10-OUNCE BOX COUSCOUS

1 CUP DICED TOMATOES

1 CUP SLICED GREEN ONION

¼ CUP CHOPPED FRESH BASIL

2 TEASPOONS MINCED GARLIC

¼ CUP BALSAMIC VINEGAR

½ CUP EXTRA-VIRGIN OLIVE OIL

SALT AND PEPPER TO TASTE

1. Bring the chicken stock to a boil in a small saucepan. Stir in the couscous in a steady stream and remove from the heat. Cover and let stand for 5 minutes until the couscous absorbs the liquid. Fluff with a fork.

2. Transfer the couscous to a large bowl and add the tomatoes, green onion, basil, and garlic.

3. In a small bowl, whisk together the vinegar and oil. Add to the salad and toss well. Season with salt and pepper to taste and refrigerate until ready to serve.

Herbed Quinoa and Arugula Salad

SERVES 4 TO 6

- ▶ PREP TIME: 10 MINUTES
- ▶ COOK TIME: 15 MINUTES

Tossed with a light, tangy dressing and studded with fresh tomatoes and red onion, this herbed quinoa salad is tender, flavorful, and packed with protein.

1 CUP QUINOA, RINSED AND DRAINED

2 CUPS WATER

2 CUPS ARUGULA

1 CUP GRAPE TOMATOES, HALVED

2 TABLESPOONS DICED RED ONION

1 GARLIC CLOVE, MINCED

2 TABLESPOONS CHOPPED FRESH CILANTRO

1 TABLESPOON CHOPPED FRESH PARSLEY

¼ CUP FRESH LIME JUICE

2 TABLESPOONS EXTRA-VIRGIN OLIVE OIL

SALT AND PEPPER TO TASTE

1. Combine the quinoa and water in a small saucepan and bring to a boil. Reduce heat and simmer, covered, for 12 to 15 minutes, until the liquid has been absorbed. Remove from heat and let sit for 5 minutes.

2. In a large serving bowl, combine the arugula, tomatoes, and red onion.

3. Whisk together the garlic, cilantro, parsley, lime juice, olive oil, and salt and pepper in a small bowl. Add to the arugula and tomatoes and toss.

4. Fluff the quinoa with a fork and add it to the other salad ingredients, tossing to mix. Serve warm.

Spinach Quinoa Salad

- ▶ PREP TIME: 5 MINUTES
- ▶ COOK TIME: 5 MINUTES

This warm, fortifying salad is perfect for a wintry day. Quinoa supplies protein, while spinach packs plenty of iron.

1 TABLESPOON EXTRA-VIRGIN OLIVE OIL

1 TEASPOON MINCED GARLIC

2 CUPS COOKED QUINOA

4 CUPS BABY SPINACH, PACKED

1½ CUPS GRAPE TOMATOES, HALVED

¼ CUP THIN-SLICED RED ONION

SALT AND PEPPER TO TASTE

2 TABLESPOONS FRESH LEMON JUICE

½ TEASPOON DRIED BASIL

¼ TEASPOON DRIED OREGANO

1. Heat the oil in a skillet over medium heat. Add the garlic and cook for 1 minute.

2. Stir in the cooked quinoa and baby spinach.

3. Add the tomatoes and onion and stir to combine. Season with salt and pepper to taste.

4. Stir in the lemon juice, basil, and oregano and cook until the spinach begins to wilt, about 2 to 3 minutes.

5. Transfer to a serving bowl and serve warm.

Warm Potato Salad

▶ PREP TIME: 15 MINUTES
▶ COOK TIME: 15 MINUTES

A twist on a traditional cold potato salad, this warm version includes sweet potatoes as well as red ones, and some shaved Parmesan.

8 RED POTATOES, QUARTERED
1 SWEET POTATO, CHOPPED
3 TABLESPOONS MAYONNAISE WITH OLIVE OIL
1 TABLESPOON EXTRA-VIRGIN OLIVE OIL
1 TABLESPOON FRESH LEMON JUICE
2 TEASPOONS ONION POWDER
1½ TEASPOONS GARLIC POWDER
SALT AND PEPPER TO TASTE
¼ CUP SHAVED PARMESAN CHEESE

1. Place the red potatoes in a large saucepan and cover them with 2 inches of cold water.

2. Bring the water to boil, then add the sweet potato. Return to a boil and cook for about 12 minutes more, or until tender, but not mushy.

3. Drain the potatoes and transfer to a large bowl.

4. In a small bowl, whisk together the mayonnaise, olive oil, lemon juice, onion powder, garlic powder, and salt and pepper. Spoon the dressing over the potatoes and toss well to coat.

5. Add the shaved Parmesan cheese, toss, and serve.

Greek Chicken Salad

SERVES 4

▶ PREP TIME: 10 MINUTES

In this chopped salad with Greek flavors, you can enjoy a little bit of every-thing—tomatoes, onion, olives, feta, and of course, chicken—in each bite.

SALAD

12 OUNCES COOKED CHICKEN, SHREDDED

6 CUPS CHOPPED ROMAINE LETTUCE

1 CUP CHOPPED TOMATOES

½ CUP THINLY SLICED RED ONION

½ CUP SLICED BLACK OLIVES

½ CUP CRUMBLED FETA CHEESE

DRESSING

¼ CUP RED WINE VINEGAR

2 TABLESPOONS EXTRA-VIRGIN OLIVE OIL

1 TABLESPOON CHOPPED FRESH DILL

1 GARLIC CLOVE, MINCED

SALT AND PEPPER TO TASTE

1. Combine the chicken, lettuce, tomatoes, onion, black olives, and feta in a salad bowl. Toss well to combine.

2. To make the dressing, whisk together the vinegar, olive oil, dill, garlic, and salt and pepper in a small bowl.

3. Add the dressing to the salad and toss well. Refrigerate until ready to serve.

Mediterranean Tuna Salad

SERVES 4

▶ PREP TIME: 10 MINUTES

Serve this tuna salad on a bed of chopped lettuce, or stuff into a pita pocket to make a sandwich.

SALAD

TWO 6-OUNCE CANS TUNA IN WATER, DRAINED

1 CUP DICED TOMATOES

1 CUCUMBER, DICED

¼ CUP DICED RED ONION

1 CUP SLICED KALAMATA OLIVES

DRESSING

2 TABLESPOONS EXTRA-VIRGIN OLIVE OIL

1 TABLESPOON RED WINE VINEGAR

1 TEASPOON DRIED OREGANO

½ TEASPOON SUGAR

SALT AND PEPPER TO TASTE

1. Flake the tuna into a large bowl and stir in the tomatoes, cucumber, red onion, and olives.

2. To make the dressing, whisk together the olive oil, vinegar, oregano, sugar, salt, and pepper in a small bowl.

3. Add the dressing to the tuna and vegetables and toss. Cover with plastic wrap and refrigerate until ready to serve.

Salmon and Orzo Salad

SERVES 4

▶ PREP TIME: 15 MINUTES

Salmon is rich in omega-3 fatty acids, a very healthful kind of fat. In this recipe, salmon is paired with onion, raisins, mint, and orzo—a type of pasta shaped like grains of rice—for a satisfying salad.

12 OUNCES UNCOOKED ORZO PASTA

¼ CUP LEMON JUICE

TWO 6-OUNCE CANS ALASKAN SALMON, DRAINED

1 CUP THINLY SLICED RED ONION

½ CUP GOLDEN RAISINS

⅓ CUP EXTRA-VIRGIN OLIVE OIL

2 TABLESPOONS CHOPPED FRESH MINT

SALT AND PEPPER TO TASTE

1. Cook the orzo according to the package directions until al dente, drain, and set aside to cool.

2. Transfer the orzo to a large bowl and toss with the lemon juice.

3. Flake the salmon into the bowl with the orzo and add the onion, raisins, olive oil, and mint. Toss, season with salt and pepper, and toss again.

4. Refrigerate until ready to serve.

CHAPTER SIX

Entrées

Linguine in Garlicky Tomato Sauce

SERVES 4

▶ PREP TIME: 15 MINUTES
▶ COOK TIME: 10 MINUTES

The flavorful red sauce with fresh herbs and plenty of garlic is easy to prepare. Double or triple the recipe for a crowd.

8 OUNCES WHOLE-GRAIN LINGUINE
2 TABLESPOONS EXTRA-VIRGIN OLIVE OIL
1 TABLESPOON MINCED GARLIC
2 CUPS CHOPPED TOMATOES
2 TABLESPOONS CHOPPED FRESH PARSLEY
2 TABLESPOONS CHOPPED FRESH BASIL
SALT AND PEPPER TO TASTE

1. Bring a pot of salted water to a boil and add the linguine. Cook according to the package directions until al dente, drain, and set aside.

2. Heat the oil in a large skillet over medium-high heat. Add the garlic and cook for 1 minute.

3. Stir in the tomatoes, parsley, and basil and season with salt and pepper. Cook, stirring, for 5 minutes.

4. Add the drained linguine to the tomatoes, stir until heated through, and serve hot.

Broccoli Rabe with Penne

SERVES 6

▶ PREP TIME: 15 MINUTES
▶ COOK TIME: 10 MINUTES

Also called rapini, broccoli rabe has a bold flavor with a slightly bitter edge. It contains high levels of glucosinolates, which are organic compounds that help prevent cancer.

12 OUNCES WHOLE-WHEAT PENNE PASTA

1 POUND BROCCOLI RABE, TRIMMED AND CHOPPED

3 TABLESPOONS EXTRA-VIRGIN OLIVE OIL

2 TABLESPOONS MINCED GARLIC

SALT AND PEPPER TO TASTE

1. Bring a large pot of salted water to boil and add the penne. Cook according to the package directions until al dente, drain, and set aside.

2. Meanwhile, bring a medium saucepan of salted water to a boil. Cook the broccoli rabe for 3 to 5 minutes, until tender, and drain.

3. Heat the oil in a large skillet over medium heat. Add the garlic and cook for 1 minute, stirring. Add the broccoli rabe and penne, and stir together with salt and pepper. Cook for 2 minutes, until heated through.

4. Serve immediately.

Chickpea Burgers with Tahini

SERVES 4

▶ PREP TIME: 10 MINUTES
▶ COOK TIME: 10 MINUTES

Also known as garbanzo beans, chickpeas are a great vegetarian source of protein and of fiber. They are eaten in Mediterranean countries in stews and soups and in that well-known dip, hummus.

BURGERS

ONE 15-OUNCE CAN CHICKPEAS, RINSED AND DRAINED

¼ CUP SLICED GREEN ONIONS

1 EGG

2 TABLESPOONS WHOLE-WHEAT FLOUR

1 TABLESPOON CHOPPED FRESH OREGANO

SALT AND PEPPER TO TASTE

2 TABLESPOONS EXTRA-VIRGIN OLIVE OIL

SAUCE

½ CUP PLAIN GREEK YOGURT

2 TABLESPOONS TAHINI (SESAME SEED PASTE)

1 TABLESPOON FRESH LEMON JUICE

PINCH OF SALT

1. Combine the chickpeas, green onions, egg, flour, and oregano in a food processor. Season with salt and pepper.

2. Process until the ingredients form a coarse mixture that starts to hold together. Remove from the food processor and shape into 4 even patties.

3. Heat the oil in a large skillet over medium-high heat. Add the patties and cook for 4 minutes on the first side until lightly browned. Carefully flip the patties and cook for 2 to 3 minutes more, until browned on the second side.

4. To make the sauce, whisk together the yogurt, tahini, and lemon juice in a small bowl and season with a pinch of salt.

5. Serve the burgers hot, topped with the sauce.

Cilantro Black Bean Burgers

SERVES 6

▶ PREP TIME: 5 MINUTES
▶ COOK TIME: 10 MINUTES

Black beans are an excellent source of vegetarian protein and fiber. In this recipe, they also make a tasty burger!

ONE 15-OUNCE CAN BLACK BEANS, RINSED AND DRAINED
1 EGG
1 CUP DICED ONION
1 CUP WHOLE-WHEAT BREAD CRUMBS
¼ CUP CHOPPED FRESH CILANTRO
SALT AND PEPPER TO TASTE
2 TABLESPOONS CANOLA OIL

1. Put the beans in a large bowl and mash lightly with a fork. Stir in the egg, onion, bread crumbs, cilantro, salt, and pepper. Stir well and shape the mixture into 6 even patties.

2. Heat the oil in a large skillet over medium-heat. Add the patties and cook for 5 minutes on the first side. Flip the patties and cook for another 5 minutes on the second side, or until heated through.

3. Serve immediately with your favorite burger toppings.

Agave Glazed Salmon

SERVES 4

- ▶ PREP TIME: 5 MINUTES
- ▶ COOK TIME: 15 MINUTES

Agave nectar is a natural sweetener made from the agave plant. In this recipe it balances the tart lime juice, giving the salmon a slightly sweet flavor.

VEGETABLE OIL FOR GRATE

FOUR 5- TO 6-OUNCE SALMON FILLETS

SALT AND PEPPER TO TASTE

⅓ CUP EXTRA-VIRGIN OLIVE OIL

⅓ CUP AGAVE NECTAR

2 TABLESPOONS LIME JUICE

1. Build a medium-hot fire in a charcoal grill or heat a gas grill to medium-high. Oil the grate.

2. Rinse the fish well in cool water and pat dry. Season with salt and pepper.

3. Whisk together the olive oil, agave nectar, and lime juice and brush some over the salmon.

4. Place the fillets on the grill and cook for 3 to 4 minutes on the first side until lightly charred. Carefully flip the fillets and brush again with the agave mixture. Grill for another 3 to 4 minutes, until the salmon is cooked through.

5. Transfer the salmon to plates and serve hot.

Herb-Crusted Tilapia Fillets

SERVES 6

▶ PREP TIME: 10 MINUTES
▶ COOK TIME: 15 MINUTES

Tender and flavorful, this tilapia recipe is the perfect dish to enjoy on the Mediterranean diet. Though high in protein, it is low in fat.

SIX 6-OUNCE TILAPIA FILLETS
3 TABLESPOONS EXTRA-VIRGIN OLIVE OIL, PLUS EXTRA
    FOR BRUSHING THE FISH
SALT AND PEPPER TO TASTE
1 CUP FRESH SPINACH LEAVES, CHOPPED
1 CUP PLAIN BREAD CRUMBS
1 TABLESPOON ITALIAN SEASONING

1. Preheat the oven to 400°F and line a baking sheet with foil.

2. Rinse the fish with cool water and pat dry. Brush with olive oil and season with salt and pepper. Place fish on the baking sheet.

3. Combine the spinach, the 3 tablespoons of olive oil, the bread crumbs, and Italian seasoning in a medium bowl.

4. Spoon about 1 tablespoon of the mixture onto each fillet and press it lightly into the fish.

5. Bake fish for 10 to 12 minutes, or until the flesh flakes easily with a fork. Serve immediately.

Fish and Tomato Packet

SERVES 4

▶ PREP TIME: 15 MINUTES
▶ COOK TIME: 15 MINUTES

This recipe is quick to throw together and it's easy to clean up, too. The foil packet holds on to the juices, keeping the fish exceptionally moist and flavorful.

VEGETABLE OIL FOR GRATE

FOUR 4- TO 5-OUNCE HALIBUT FILLETS, OR ANOTHER FIRM-FLESHED FISH

2 TABLESPOONS LEMON JUICE

SALT AND PEPPER TO TASTE

4 CUPS CHOPPED SPINACH

2 CUPS COARSELY CHOPPED TOMATOES

1 ONION, CHOPPED

1 TABLESPOON MINCED GARLIC

¼ CUP BALSAMIC VINEGAR

2 TABLESPOONS EXTRA-VIRGIN OLIVE OIL

2 TABLESPOONS CHOPPED FRESH BASIL

1. Build a medium-hot fire in a charcoal grill or heat a gas grill to medium-high. Oil the grate.

2. Rinse the fish well in cool water and pat dry. Place the fish on a foil-lined platter. Brush the lemon juice over the fish and season with salt and pepper.

3. Combine the spinach, tomatoes, onion, and garlic in a large mixing bowl. Add balsamic vinegar, olive oil, and basil and stir to combine.

4. Spoon the spinach mixture over the fish and cover the fish with a second piece of foil. Fold over and crimp the edges of the foil to create a packet. Carefully slide the packet off the plate and onto the grill.

5. Cover the grill and cook for 15 minutes or until the fish is cooked through. Serve hot.

Easy Shrimp Scampi with Spaghetti

SERVES 6

▶ PREP TIME: 15 MINUTES
▶ COOK TIME: 10 MINUTES

Shrimp scampi is traditionally made with butter, but this recipe uses a combination of olive oil and butter substitute to reduce the calorie and saturated fat content of the dish. Olive-oil-based butter substitute works especially well.

8 OUNCES WHOLE-WHEAT SPAGHETTI

2 TABLESPOONS EXTRA-VIRGIN OLIVE OIL

2 POUNDS RAW SHRIMP, PEELED AND DEVEINED

1 TABLESPOON MINCED GARLIC

¼ CUP DICED SHALLOTS

2 TABLESPOONS FRESH LEMON JUICE

2 TABLESPOONS DRY SHERRY

3 TABLESPOONS CHOPPED FRESH PARSLEY

SALT AND PEPPER TO TASTE

3 TABLESPOONS BUTTER SUBSTITUTE

1. Bring a pot of salted water to boil and add the spaghetti. Cook according to the package directions until al dente, drain, and transfer to a large bowl. Keep warm.

2. Heat the olive oil in a large skillet over medium heat. Add the shrimp and cook for 3 minutes without stirring. Turn the shrimp and cook for 1 to 2 minutes on the other side until cooked through. Transfer the shrimp to a bowl and keep warm.

3. Stir the garlic and shallots into the skillet and cook for 30 seconds. Add the lemon juice, sherry, and parsley. Season with salt and pepper and stir well.

4. Remove from the heat and add the cooked shrimp and butter substitute to the pan. Toss to coat the shrimp and let sit for 2 minutes.

5. Divide the spaghetti among six plates and spoon the shrimp on top.

Grilled Lemon Garlic Swordfish

▶ PREP TIME: 10 MINUTES
▶ COOK TIME: 10 MINUTES

Swordfish has a dense and meaty texture, which pairs well with the fresh taste of lemon juice. The fish is not only incredibly flavorful, but also a good source of omega-3 fatty acids as well as protein.

VEGETABLE OIL FOR GRATE
FOUR 6-OUNCE SWORDFISH STEAKS
SALT AND PEPPER TO TASTE
3 TABLESPOONS LEMON JUICE
2 TABLESPOONS EXTRA-VIRGIN OLIVE OIL
1 TABLESPOON MINCED GARLIC

1. Build a hot fire in a charcoal grill or heat a gas grill to high. Oil the grate.

2. Rinse the fish well in cool water and pat dry. Season with salt and pepper.

3. Whisk together the lemon juice, olive oil, and garlic in a small bowl.

4. Brush the lemon mixture onto both sides of the fish and place on the grill. Cook for 4 minutes on the first side. Carefully turn the fish and brush again with the lemon mixture.

5. Grill for another 4 minutes, or until the flesh flakes easily with a fork. Serve hot.

Chicken Shawarma Pita Pockets

SERVES 4

▶ PREP TIME: 15 MINUTES
▶ COOK TIME: 10 MINUTES

Middle Eastern shawarma is similar to Greek gyro. Spiced meat is molded around the spit on which it cooks, and portions are shaved off and eaten with flatbread. In this adaptation, thinly sliced chicken is tucked into pita bread along with a savory yogurt sauce.

¼ CUP PLUS 1 TABLESPOON PLAIN GREEK YOGURT

2 TABLESPOONS FRESH LEMON JUICE

1 TEASPOON MINCED GARLIC

1 TABLESPOON TAHINI

FOUR 6-INCH PITA BREADS, HALVED CROSSWISE

2 TABLESPOONS CHOPPED FRESH PARSLEY

¼ TEASPOON GROUND GINGER

¼ TEASPOON GROUND CORIANDER

SALT AND PEPPER TO TASTE

1 POUND BONELESS SKINLESS CHICKEN, THINLY SLICED

1 TABLESPOON EXTRA-VIRGIN OLIVE OIL

½ CUP DICED CUCUMBER

½ CUP DICED TOMATO

¼ CUP THINLY SLICED RED ONION

1. Stir together ¼ cup of the yogurt, 1 tablespoon of the lemon juice, garlic, and tahini in a small bowl. Spread the mixture evenly inside each of the pita halves, and set aside.

continued ▶

2. Stir together the parsley, ginger, coriander, salt, pepper, and the remaining 1 tablespoon each of yogurt and lemon juice in a medium shallow bowl. Add the chicken and toss to coat.

3. Heat the oil in a skillet over medium-high heat. Add the chicken and cook for 6 to 8 minutes, stirring, until cooked through.

4. Spoon the chicken into the pita halves and top with cucumber, tomato, and red onion. Serve immediately.

Balsamic Chicken with Peppers

SERVES 4

▶ PREP TIME: 10 MINUTES
▶ COOK TIME: 15 MINUTES

This dish is a snap to throw together. After just a short time in the oven, the chicken emerges tender and flavorful. Feel free to prepare it in advance and refrigerate. Before serving, just rewarm for 10 to 15 minutes in the oven.

2 RED BELL PEPPERS, SLICED

1 GREEN BELL PEPPER, SLICED

1 YELLOW BELL PEPPER, SLICED

1 ONION, SLICED

⅓ CUP BALSAMIC VINEGAR

¼ CUP EXTRA-VIRGIN OLIVE OIL

¼ CUP CHICKEN BROTH

1 TABLESPOON MINCED GARLIC

1 TABLESPOON DRIED BASIL

1 TEASPOON DRIED THYME

4 BONELESS SKINLESS CHICKEN BREAST HALVES

SALT AND PEPPER TO TASTE

1. Preheat the oven to 375°F.

2. Combine the peppers and onions in a large bowl. In a small bowl, whisk together the balsamic vinegar, olive oil, chicken broth, garlic, basil, and thyme. Pour over the peppers and onions and toss well.

3. Place the chicken breasts in a greased baking pan and season with salt and pepper. Spread the pepper and onion mixture over the tops, and cover loosely with foil.

4. Bake for 15 minutes, or until the chicken is cooked through and the peppers are tender. Serve hot.

Honey Mustard Grilled Chicken

SERVES 6

▶ PREP TIME: 10 MINUTES
▶ COOK TIME: 15 MINUTES

If you are tired of plain old grilled chicken, soak it in a honey mustard marinade for a simple and tasty change. It only takes a few minutes to cook on the grill.

¼ CUP HONEY MUSTARD
¼ CUP BALSAMIC VINEGAR
2 TABLESPOONS EXTRA-VIRGIN OLIVE OIL
1 TEASPOON MINCED GARLIC
6 BONELESS SKINLESS CHICKEN BREAST HALVES
SALT AND PEPPER TO TASTE
VEGETABLE OIL FOR GRATE

1. Whisk together the honey mustard, balsamic vinegar, olive oil, and garlic in a small bowl.

2. Season the chicken with salt and pepper and place in a shallow dish. Pour the marinade over the chicken and turn once to coat. If you have time, refrigerate for 1 to 2 hours to give the chicken a good soak in the marinade.

3. Build a medium-hot fire in a charcoal grill or heat a gas grill to medium-high. Oil the grate.

4. Place the chicken breasts on the grill and cook for 5 minutes on each side, or until cooked through. Let sit for 5 minutes before slicing and serving.

Sausage-Stuffed Tomatoes

SERVES 4

▶ PREP TIME: 15 MINUTES
▶ COOK TIME: 25 MINUTES

This hearty recipe is a delicious blend of Italian flavors, from the sausage and garlic to the ripe tomatoes.

8 OUNCES GROUND ITALIAN SAUSAGE
1 CUP COOKED BROWN RICE
1½ TABLESPOONS EXTRA-VIRGIN OLIVE OIL
½ CUP DICED RED ONION
1 TABLESPOON MINCED GARLIC
SALT AND PEPPER TO TASTE
1 TEASPOON ITALIAN SEASONING
4 TOMATOES
½ CUP CRUMBLED GOAT CHEESE

1. Preheat the oven to 375°F.

2. Heat a skillet over medium-high heat and add the sausage. Cook, breaking it up with a spoon, until browned and cooked through, about 5 minutes. Remove from the pan and transfer to a medium bowl. Add the rice and set aside.

3. After draining the fat from the skillet, heat the olive oil. Add the onion and garlic and cook over medium-high heat until tender, about 5 minutes. Stir this into the sausage mixture and season with salt, pepper, and Italian seasoning.

4. Slice the tops off the tomatoes and carefully remove the pulp and seeds to hollow them out. Place the tomatoes in a glass baking dish and stuff the sausage mixture into the tomatoes. Sprinkle goat cheese on top.

5. Pour about 1 inch of boiling water into the dish around the tomatoes. Loosely cover with foil and bake for 15 minutes, or until the stuffing is hot. Serve immediately.

Pork and Turkey Meatballs

SERVES 4

▶ PREP TIME: 10 MINUTES
▶ COOK TIME: 15 MINUTES

These meatballs are lower in saturated fat than their beefy counterparts and taste great with spaghetti in a flavorful marinara sauce.

8 OUNCES WHOLE-WHEAT SPAGHETTI

12 OUNCES LEAN GROUND TURKEY

4 OUNCES GROUND PORK

2 TABLESPOONS PLAIN BREAD CRUMBS

1 EGG

¼ CUP MINCED RED ONION

¼ CUP FRESH CHOPPED PARSLEY

2 TABLESPOONS FRESH CHOPPED CHIVES

SALT AND PEPPER TO TASTE

1 TABLESPOON EXTRA-VIRGIN OLIVE OIL

2 CUPS PREPARED MARINARA SAUCE

1. Bring a pot of salted water to a boil. Cook the spaghetti in the boiling water according to the package directions until al dente. Drain and keep warm in a large bowl.

2. Meanwhile, combine the ground turkey and pork, bread crumbs, egg, red onion, parsley, chives, salt, and pepper in a large mixing bowl. Mix to combine well and shape by hand into 1½-inch balls.

3. Heat the oil in a large sauté pan over high heat. Add the meatballs and cook for 3 to 5 minutes, turning often, until evenly browned.

4. Pour in the marinara sauce, reduce the heat and simmer for 10 minutes, or until the meatballs are cooked through.

5. Add the meatballs and sauce to the spaghetti. Toss and serve.

Easy Lamb Kofta

SERVES 4

▶ PREP TIME: 10 MINUTES
▶ COOK TIME: 10 MINUTES

Variations of lamb kofta are eaten in Turkey and around the Middle East. Sometimes they're made into meatballs, and sometimes, as in this Turkish version, they are shaped into patties. The yogurt sauce makes a perfect accompaniment.

YOGURT SAUCE

1 CUP PLAIN GREEK YOGURT
3 TABLESPOONS CHOPPED FRESH MINT
1 TABLESPOON FRESH LEMON JUICE
1 GARLIC CLOVE, MINCED

LAMB KOFTA

1 POUND GROUND LAMB
1 EGG, LIGHTLY BEATEN
½ CUP MINCED RED ONION
¼ CUP CHOPPED FRESH PARSLEY
½ TEASPOON GROUND CUMIN
¼ TEASPOON GROUND CINNAMON
SALT AND PEPPER TO TASTE
1 TABLESPOON EXTRA-VIRGIN OLIVE OIL

1. Stir together the yogurt, mint, lemon juice, and garlic in a small bowl. Set aside.

2. Combine the lamb, egg, onion, parsley, cumin, cinnamon, salt, and pepper in a mixing bowl and stir well. Shape the mixture into 2-inch balls and flatten into patties by hand.

3. Heat the olive oil in a large skillet over medium-high heat. Add the patties and cook for 3 minutes on the first side. Flip the patties and cook for another 2 minutes on the second side, or until cooked through.

4. Drain the kofta on paper towels and serve warm with the yogurt sauce.

Rosemary Lamb Chops

SERVES 4

▶ PREP TIME: 5 MINUTES
▶ COOK TIME: 10 MINUTES

If you are looking for a quick and satisfying meal, these rosemary lamb chops are the way to go. Simply season them as you see fit and broil to the desired level of doneness.

EIGHT 4-OUNCE BONE-IN LAMB CHOPS
SALT AND PEPPER TO TASTE
1 TABLESPOON MINCED GARLIC
2 TEASPOONS DRIED ROSEMARY
1 TEASPOON DRIED OREGANO

1. Preheat the broiler.

2. Season the chops with salt and pepper. Combine the garlic, rosemary, and oregano in a small bowl and rub the mixture into the chops on both sides.

3. Place the chops in a broiler pan and broil for 4 minutes on each side, or until cooked to the desired level of doneness. Serve hot.

Pomegranate Beef Tips

SERVES 4

▶ PREP TIME: 10 MINUTES
▶ COOK TIME: 15 MINUTES

You may not see pomegranate juice and beef together very often, but in this recipe, they are perfectly matched. The juice is packed with healthful antioxidants—an added bonus.

1 TABLESPOON EXTRA-VIRGIN OLIVE OIL

1½ POUNDS BEEF SIRLOIN, CHOPPED

1 TEASPOON MINCED GARLIC

1 ONION, CHOPPED

ONE 14-OUNCE CAN CRUSHED TOMATOES

1 CUP UNSWEETENED POMEGRANATE JUICE

¼ CUP BALSAMIC VINEGAR

2 TABLESPOONS HONEY

½ CUP GOLDEN RAISINS

SALT AND PEPPER TO TASTE

1. Heat the olive oil in a large skillet over medium-high heat. Add the beef and brown for 2 minutes, stirring often. Stir in the garlic and cook for 1 minute.

2. Add the tomatoes, pomegranate juice, balsamic vinegar, honey, raisins, salt, and pepper. Stir well to combine.

3. Bring the mixture to a simmer, lower the heat, and cook, covered, for 10 minutes or until the beef is tender. Serve hot.

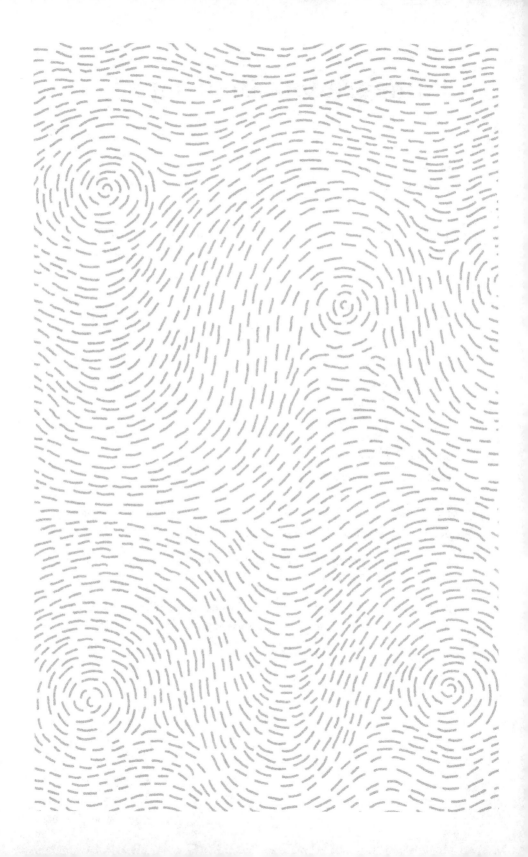

CHAPTER SEVEN

Desserts and Drinks

Cinnamon Spice Cookies

MAKES 3 DOZEN COOKIES

▶ PREP TIME: 15 MINUTES
▶ COOK TIME: 15 MINUTES

Spiced with cinnamon and hints of mace and cloves, these cookies are soft and sweet, with a little bit of bite. Note that the cookie dough needs to rest in the refrigerator overnight.

¾ CUP EXTRA-VIRGIN OLIVE OIL

¼ CUP MOLASSES

1¼ CUPS SUGAR

2 EGGS

1 TEASPOON ALMOND EXTRACT

1¾ CUPS ALL-PURPOSE FLOUR

1 CUP WHOLE-WHEAT FLOUR

1½ TEASPOONS BAKING SODA

1½ TABLESPOONS GROUND CINNAMON

1 TABLESPOON GROUND GINGER

1 TEASPOON GROUND MACE

1 TEASPOON GROUND CLOVES

½ TEASPOON SALT

1. Beat together the olive oil, molasses, 1 cup of the sugar, eggs, and almond extract in a large mixing bowl.

2. In a separate bowl, whisk together the flours, baking soda, cinnamon, ginger, mace, cloves, and salt.

3. Add the dry ingredients to the wet, and whisk until well combined. Cover and chill overnight.

4. Preheat oven to 350°F and line two baking sheets with parchment paper.

5. Put the remaining ¼ cup of sugar in a shallow dish. Pinch off pieces of dough and roll them into 1½-inch balls. Roll the balls in the sugar; then arrange them on the baking sheets.

6. Bake for 10 to 12 minutes, or until the tops just begin to crack. Cool on the pans for 5 minutes, transfer to wire racks, and cool completely.

Italian Anise Cookies

MAKES 3 DOZEN COOKIES

▶ PREP TIME: 15 MINUTES
▶ COOK TIME: 10 MINUTES

Anise seeds come from a flowering plant native to the eastern Mediterranean region. These small, delicious cookies make the most of its unique flavor, in the form of anise extract.

4 CUPS ALL-PURPOSE FLOUR
1 CUP SUGAR
1 TABLESPOON BAKING POWDER
¼ TEASPOON SALT
2 EGGS
¾ CUP VEGETABLE OIL
½ CUP MILK
1 TABLESPOON ANISE EXTRACT

1. Preheat the oven to 350°F. Line two baking sheets with parchment paper.

2. Whisk together the flour, sugar, baking powder, and salt in a large mixing bowl.

3. In a medium bowl, whisk together the eggs, oil, milk, and anise extract until smooth.

4. Make a well in the center of the dry ingredients and pour in the wet ingredients. Work the mixture into a dough by hand. Dough will be sticky.

5. Oil your hands to keep dough from sticking. Roll dough into 1-inch balls and arrange them on the baking sheets, flattening the balls slightly.

6. Bake for 8 minutes, until just starting to brown. Cool on wire racks.

Avocado Oatmeal Cookies

MAKES 2 DOZEN COOKIES

▶ PREP TIME: 15 MINUTES
▶ COOK TIME: 15 MINUTES

Avocado may sound like a strange ingredient for a baked good, but it's what makes these cookies moist and flavorful—everything you could ask for in a cookie! For your convenience, feel free to prepare the dough several days ahead and store it in the refrigerator until you are ready to bake.

1 CUP ALL-PURPOSE FLOUR

½ TEASPOON BAKING SODA

½ TEASPOON BAKING POWDER

PINCH OF SALT

½ CUP (1 STICK) UNSALTED BUTTER, AT ROOM TEMPERATURE

½ CUP PACKED LIGHT BROWN SUGAR

¼ CUP GRANULATED SUGAR

1 EGG

1 RIPE AVOCADO, PITTED, SKIN REMOVED, AND MASHED

1½ CUPS ROLLED (OLD-FASHIONED) OATS

1. Preheat the oven to 325°F. Line two baking sheets with parchment paper.

2. Sift the flour, baking soda, baking powder, and salt into a medium bowl and set aside.

3. With an electric mixer, beat the butter in a large mixing bowl until creamy; then beat in the brown and white sugars. Scrape down the sides of the bowl. Add the egg and beat on high speed until well combined. Add the avocado, beating just until incorporated.

4. With the mixer on low speed, gradually add the oats and then the flour mixture, beating just until combined.

continued ▶

5. Spoon the batter onto the prepared baking sheets in heaping tablespoons, and flatten each cookie slightly.

6. Bake the cookies for 15 minutes or until lightly browned. Transfer to a wire rack to cool.

Avocado Sorbet

SERVES 4

▶ PREP TIME: 5 MINUTES
▶ COOK TIME: 10 MINUTES

You still may not think of avocado as a dessert item, but after trying this refreshing sorbet, you are sure to become a believer. Avocados contain monounsaturated fat, like the fat in olive oil, which is a good source of antioxidants.

1 CUP WATER
¼ CUP SUGAR
2 RIPE AVOCADOS, PITTED AND SKIN REMOVED
2 TABLESPOONS LIME JUICE
1 TEASPOON GRATED LIME ZEST
1 TABLESPOON HONEY

1. Whisk together the water and sugar in a small saucepan over medium heat. Cook, whisking often, until the sugar dissolves, about 2 minutes. Remove from the heat and cool.

2. Put the avocadoes in a food processor. Pour in the sugar water and add the lime juice, lime zest, and honey. Process until smooth and transfer to a metal baking pan, spreading out the mixture evenly.

3. Cover with aluminum foil and freeze until solid.

4. When ready to serve, break the sorbet into pieces, and pulse in a food processor until smooth. Spoon into dessert dishes.

Peach Nectarine Granita

SERVES 4

▶ PREP TIME: 10 MINUTES
▶ COOK TIME: 15 MINUTES

This refreshing granita is the perfect way to enjoy fresh summer fruit. Feel free to substitute plums for the nectarines and peaches, or use a combination of all three.

1 CUP SLICED, PEELED RIPE PEACHES
1 CUP SLICED, PEELED RIPE NECTARINES
½ CUP SUGAR
½ CUP WATER
½ CUP FRESH RASPBERRIES
¼ CUP FRESH ORANGE JUICE
2 TABLESPOONS FRESH LEMON JUICE

1. In a large saucepan, combine the peaches, nectarines, sugar, and water over medium-high heat. Bring the mixture to a boil, reduce the heat, and simmer, covered, for 10 minutes. Remove from the heat and stir in the raspberries.

2. Pour the fruit mixture into a blender and blend until smooth. Strain through a mesh sieve into a mixing bowl and discard the pulp.

3. Stir in the orange juice and lemon juice. Pour into a shallow baking pan and cover with aluminum foil.

4. Freeze the mixture until ice crystals form around the edges, about 30 minutes. Stir, moving the ice crystals toward the center of the pan, and freeze for another 30 minutes. Repeat the process once or twice more until frozen solid, with a grainy texture.

5. Break the granita up with a knife and serve.

Plum Caprese Salad

SERVES 8

▶ PREP TIME: 10 MINUTES
▶ COOK TIME: 15 MINUTES

Traditional caprese salad is made with fresh tomatoes and mozzarella. When you replace the tomatoes with ripe plums and drizzle them with a pomegranate syrup, the salad becomes a light and refreshing dessert. This is also good with rounds of goat cheese.

½ CUP UNSWEETENED POMEGRANATE JUICE
2 TABLESPOONS BALSAMIC VINEGAR
1 TEASPOON SUGAR
2 RIPE PURPLE PLUMS, PITTED AND THINLY SLICED
1 RIPE GREEN PLUM, PITTED AND THINLY SLICED
8 OUNCES FRESH MOZZARELLA, THINLY SLICED
2 TABLESPOONS EXTRA-VIRGIN OLIVE OIL
2 TABLESPOONS CHOPPED FRESH BASIL

1. Pour the pomegranate juice into a small saucepan and bring to a simmer. Cook, whisking occasionally, for 10 minutes, or until syrupy and reduced to about 2 tablespoons. Whisk in the balsamic vinegar and sugar. Transfer to a small bowl, cover, and refrigerate until ready to serve.

2. Arrange the plum and mozzarella slices on a platter, alternating between the two.

3. Drizzle the pomegranate mixture over the plums. Drizzle with olive oil, sprinkle with basil, and serve.

Baked Stuffed Pears

SERVES 8

▶ PREP TIME: 15 MINUTES
▶ COOK TIME: 20 MINUTES

This recipe is the perfect combination of tender pears and crunchy walnuts, sure to please.

1¼ CUPS SUGAR
¾ CUP WATER
⅛ TEASPOON CREAM OF TARTAR
8 RIPE PEARS, PEELED
1 CUP APPLE JUICE
½ CUP RAISINS
⅓ CUP CHOPPED WALNUTS
2 TABLESPOONS LEMON JUICE

1. Preheat the oven to 350°F.

2. Whisk together 1 cup of the sugar, ¼ cup of the water, and the cream of tartar in a large saucepan. Bring to a boil, stirring often. Reduce the heat, cover, and cook for 3 minutes. Uncover and let the syrup simmer over low heat until thickened. Set aside.

3. Meanwhile, cut the pears in half lengthwise and scoop out the cores. Place the pears in a microwave-safe dish, cut side down, and pour the apple juice in the dish around them. Microwave on high for 3 minutes, or until they begin to soften.

4. Combine the raisins, walnuts, the remaining ¼ cup sugar, and the lemon juice in a small bowl and stir well.

5. Transfer the pears to a baking dish, cut side up, and spoon the raisin-walnut mixture into the cavities.

6. Whisk the remaining ½ cup of water into the syrup and pour it into the baking dish, around the pears.

7. Cover the pears with aluminum foil and bake for 15 minutes, or until the pears are tender and the filling hot. Serve.

Apricots with Yogurt and Honey

SERVES 2

▶ PREP TIME: 5 MINUTES

Fresh apricots need very little—some yogurt, a drizzle of honey, and some chopped pistachios—and you have yourself an excellent dessert. These slightly tart little stone fruits are full of vitamin C and beta-carotene.

2 RIPE APRICOTS, PITTED AND HALVED

¼ CUP PLAIN GREEK YOGURT

2 TABLESPOONS WILDFLOWER HONEY

2 TABLESPOONS SHELLED PISTACHIOS, CHOPPED

1. Divide the apricots between two small bowls and top each serving with 2 tablespoons yogurt.

2. Drizzle the apricots with the honey, sprinkle pistachios on top, and serve.

Figs in Balsamic Syrup

SERVES 6

▶ PREP TIME: 15 MINUTES
▶ COOK TIME: 15 MINUTES

Figs are a good source of potassium, which helps to lower and control blood pressure. Dried Mission figs are purplish-black and contain tiny seeds.

1 CUP DRY RED WINE
¼ CUP BALSAMIC VINEGAR
½ CUP SUGAR
1 POUND DRIED MISSION FIGS, STEMMED
2 TABLESPOONS CHOPPED WALNUTS

1. Preheat the oven to 350°F.

2. Whisk together the wine, vinegar, and sugar in a medium saucepan over medium heat. Cook, whisking often, until the sugar dissolves. Add the figs and bring to a simmer. Lower the heat, cover, and simmer for 5 minutes.

3. Transfer the figs and liquid to a shallow baking dish and sprinkle with the walnuts. Bake, covered, for 15 minutes or until the figs are softened.

4. Cool the figs for 10 minutes and serve.

Spiced Fruit Compote

SERVES 6

▶ PREP TIME: 5 MINUTES
▶ COOK TIME: 15 MINUTES

This compote is absolutely delicious on its own or spooned over a bowl of vanilla ice cream or Greek yogurt. The compote needs to sit in the refrigerator for at least 6 hours to marry the flavors.

1 SPRIG FRESH ROSEMARY

TWO 5-INCH STRIPS ORANGE ZEST

1 TEASPOON WHOLE PEPPERCORNS

3 CUPS FRESH ORANGE JUICE

2 CUPS DRIED APRICOTS

1 CUP GOLDEN RAISINS

½ CUP DRIED CHERRIES

¾ CUP DRY WHITE WINE

¾ CUP SUGAR

1. Place the rosemary, orange zest, and peppercorns on a square of damp cheesecloth. Wrap the cheesecloth around them and tie the packet closed to make a spice bouquet.

2. Combine the orange juice, apricots, raisins, cherries, wine, and sugar in a large saucepan over medium-high heat. Add the spice bouquet.

3. Bring to a boil, stirring until the sugar dissolves. Reduce the heat and simmer, uncovered, for 15 minutes or until the fruit is tender.

4. Remove from the heat and transfer to a bowl to cool. Remove spice bouquet. Refrigerate the compote for at least 6 hours or up to 2 days.

Maple Brown Rice Pudding

SERVES 6 TO 8

▶ PREP TIME: 5 MINUTES
▶ COOK TIME: 15 MINUTES

Warm and creamy, this brown rice pudding is simple to make and absolutely delicious.

2 CUPS COOKED BROWN RICE

3 CUPS UNSWEETENED ALMOND MILK

3 EGGS

½ CUP PACKED LIGHT BROWN SUGAR

¼ CUP PURE MAPLE SYRUP

1 TEASPOON VANILLA EXTRACT

½ TEASPOON GROUND CINNAMON

¼ TEASPOON GROUND NUTMEG

PINCH OF SALT

1. Combine all the ingredients in a large mixing bowl and stir well.

2. Spoon the mixture into a greased microwave-safe dish. Cook the mixture on high power in 2-minute increments until the center is just set, about 10 to 12 minutes total.

3. Spoon the pudding into bowls to serve.

Flourless Chocolate Cakes

SERVES 6

▶ PREP TIME: 15 MINUTES
▶ COOK TIME: 15 MINUTES

These little chocolate cakes have a rich and decadent flavor that you are sure to love. Made with olive oil instead of butter, they're exceptionally smooth and lower in saturated fat.

1½ CUPS SLIVERED ALMONDS
7 OUNCES BITTERSWEET CHOCOLATE, CHOPPED
½ CUP EXTRA-VIRGIN OLIVE OIL
5 EGGS, SEPARATED
1 CUP SUGAR
1 TABLESPOON BRANDY

1. Preheat the oven to 350°F. Grease six 7-ounce ramekins.

2. Pulse the almonds in a food processor until ground into a fine powder.

3. Melt the chocolate in the top of a double boiler over medium-low heat. Remove from the heat and whisk in the olive oil. Set aside.

4. Whisk together the egg yolks and ¾ cup of the sugar in a large mixing bowl. Beat with an electric mixer about 2 minutes.

5. Whisk in the melted chocolate mixture and the brandy and stir until smooth. Set aside.

6. In a separate large bowl, beat the egg whites with an electric mixer until soft peaks form. Add the remaining 4 tablespoons of sugar, 1 tablespoon at a time, and beat until stiff.

7. Gently fold the egg whites into the chocolate mixture until incorporated. Spoon the batter into the greased ramekins.

8. Bake for 15 minutes or so until a knife inserted in the center comes out clean. Cool in the ramekins on a wire rack before serving.

Flourless Almond Lemon Cakes

SERVES 6

▶ PREP TIME: 10 MINUTES
▶ COOK TIME: 15 MINUTES

This recipe was inspired by a traditional Majorcan dessert. It is often served with almond ice cream.

1¼ CUPS SLIVERED ALMONDS
½ CUP SUGAR
4 EGGS, SEPARATED
1 TABLESPOON GRATED LEMON ZEST
½ TEASPOON GROUND CINNAMON
PINCH OF SALT

1. Preheat the oven to 375°F and grease six 7-ounce ramekins.

2. Combine the almonds and 2 tablespoons of the sugar in a food processor and pulse until ground into a fine powder. Set aside.

3. Whisk together the egg yolks, 2 more tablespoons of the sugar, the lemon zest, cinnamon, and salt in a medium mixing bowl. Beat with an electric mixer about 2 minutes. Stir in the almond mixture.

4. In a medium bowl, beat the egg whites with an electric mixer until soft peaks form. Add the remaining ¼ cup of sugar, 1 tablespoon at a time, and beat until stiff. Gently fold the egg whites into the batter until incorporated.

5. Spoon the batter into the greased ramekins. Bake for 15 minutes or until the tip of a knife inserted in the center comes out clean. Cool on a wire rack before serving.

Hot Italian Toddy

SERVES 2

▶ PREP TIME: 5 MINUTES
▶ COOK TIME: 5 MINUTES

Tuaca is a vanilla and citrus–flavored liqueur produced in Livorno, Italy. It is what gives this wintry drink its Mediterranean flair.

2 CUPS APPLE CIDER
PINCH OF GROUND CINNAMON
2 OUNCES TUACA LIQUEUR

1. Whisk together the apple cider and cinnamon in a small saucepan. Heat the cider over medium heat until steaming. Remove from the heat and whisk in the Tuaca.

2. Pour into mugs and serve hot.

Cioccolata Calda

SERVES 2

▶ PREP TIME: 5 MINUTES
▶ COOK TIME: 10 MINUTES

Traditional Italian hot chocolate is thick and creamy—similar to pudding in consistency. Prepare this recipe and try it yourself!

1½ TABLESPOONS SUGAR
3 TABLESPOONS UNSWEETENED COCOA POWDER
1½ CUPS PLUS 2 TABLESPOONS MILK
1 TABLESPOON CORNSTARCH

1. Combine the sugar and cocoa powder in a small saucepan, and whisk in 1½ cups of the milk. Heat over medium heat until the sugar has dissolved. Reduce the heat and bring to a simmer.

2. Whisk together the remaining 2 tablespoons of milk with the cornstarch in a small bowl, then whisk into the cocoa mixture.

3. Cook the hot chocolate, whisking often, until it thickens to the consistency of pudding, about 2 to 3 minutes more. Serve hot.

Notes

Chapter One

p. 6   **Decades of medical research have shown:** Francesco Sofi, Francesca Cesari, Rosanna Abbate, et al. "Adherence to Mediterranean diet and health status: Meta-analysis." *British Medical Journal* 337 (2008): a1334. http://www.bmj.com /content/337/bmj.a1344

p. 6   **And when the Mediterranean diet is combined with moderate exercise:** Dora Romaguera, Teresa Norat, Traci Mouw, Anne M. May, Christina Bamia, Nadia Slimani, Noemie Travier, et al. "Adherence to the Mediterranean diet is associated with lower abdominal adiposity in European men and women." *Journal of Nutrition* 139, no. 9 (July 2009): 1728–37. http://www.ncbi.nlm.nih.gov/pubmed/19571036

p. 6   **A study published in the *British Medical Journal*:** Sofi et al., 2008.

p. 6   **Scientists and nutritionists have been studying the Mediterranean diet:** Anna Ferro-Luzzi and Francesco Branca. "Mediterranean diet, Italian-style: Prototype of a healthy diet." *The American Society for Clinical Nutrition* 61 (suppl.) (1995): 1338S-45S. http://ajcn.nutrition.org/content/61/6/1338S.full.pdf

Chapter Two

p. 10   **The study revealed that regular family meals:** Eliza Cook and Rachel Duniform. "Do family meals really make a difference?" *Parenting in Context* (2012), College of Human Ecology, Cornell University. http://www.human.cornell.edu/pam /outreach/upload/Family-Mealtimes-2.pdf

p. 11   **In fact, the top three income brackets:** I Love Coupon Month. "Coupon statistics." I Love Coupon Month.com. http://www.ilovecouponmonth.com/statistics

References

Eliza Cook and Rachel Duniform. "Do family meals really make a difference?" *Parenting in Context* (2012). College of Human Ecology, Cornell University. http://www.human.cornell.edu/pam/outreach/upload/Family-Mealtimes-2.pdf

Anna Ferro-Luzzi and Francesco Branca. "Mediterranean diet, Italian-style: Prototype of a healthy diet." *The American Society for Clinical Nutrition* 61 (suppl.) (1995): 1338S-45S. http://ajcn.nutrition.org/content/61/6/1338S.full.pdf

I Love Coupon Month. "Coupon statistics." I Love Coupon Month.com. http://www.ilovecouponmonth.com/statistics/

Mayo Clinic staff. "Mediterranean diet: A heart-healthy eating plan." Mayo Clinic. http://www.mayoclinic.org/mediterranean-diet/art-20047801

Mediterranean Yachting. "The Mediterranean sea: A brief history." Mediterranean -Yachting.com. http://www.mediterranean-yachting.com/History.htm

"Mediterranean diet pyramid." Oldways. http://oldwayspt.org/sites/default /files/images/Med_pyramid_flyer.jpg

"Traditional Med diet." Oldways. http://oldwayspt.org/resources/heritage -pyramids/mediterranean-diet-pyramid/traditional-med-diet

"What is the Mediterranean diet?" Oldways. http://oldwayspt.org/programs /mediterranean-foods-alliance/what-mediterranean-diet

Dora Romaguera, Teresa Norat, Traci Mouw, Anne M. May, Christina Bamia, Nadia Slimani, Noemie Travier, et al. "Adherence to the Mediterranean diet is associated with lower abdominal adiposity in European men and women." *Journal of Nutrition* 139, no. 9 (July 2009): 1728–37. http://www.ncbi.nlm.nih.gov/pubmed/19571036

Francesco Sofi, Francesca Cesari, Rosanna Abbate, et al. "Adherence to Mediterranean diet and health status: Meta-analysis." *British Medical Journal* 337 (2008): a1334. http://www.bmj.com/content/337/bmj.a1344

Index